The G.I. Diet has already helped tens of thousands of readers to lose weight!

"Following the G.I. Diet was the easiest thing I've ever done to lose weight. I went from a size 18–20 to an 8–10. It is the best gift I have ever given myself. I am 52 years young and I have more energy than ever before. Your diet changed my life—or should I say, saved it."—Bobbi

"Your diet has been a godsend to me! I weighed 195 pounds. My doctor told me I needed to go on high blood pressure medicine. I convinced her to let me try to lower my blood pressure naturally. It is now one year later and I weigh 137 pounds, my blood pressure is perfect without medicine, and I have lost approximately 40 inches. I feel so much better; I will never go back to my old, bad eating habits."—Jeri

"From a weight of 340 pounds, I now weigh exactly 196 pounds. That is a total loss in one full year of 144 pounds! I am delighted with how the G.I. Diet has changed my life. My doctor is amazed and regards my health as a complete turnaround. My life is completely different as my confidence and self-esteem have returned."—Martin

"So far, I have lost 56 pounds on the G.I. Diet. I am most satisfied with all the results so far. I don't feel deprived—I feel free."—Claire-Anne

"Your diet works like a miracle cure—it's so simple to follow. I have lost 28 pounds in 10 weeks; my husband has lost 35 pounds. I have had a birthday and numerous functions (and lost weight!) and enjoyed every minute of it. Thank you so much for your advice and inspiration. Your diet is a true revelation."—Helen

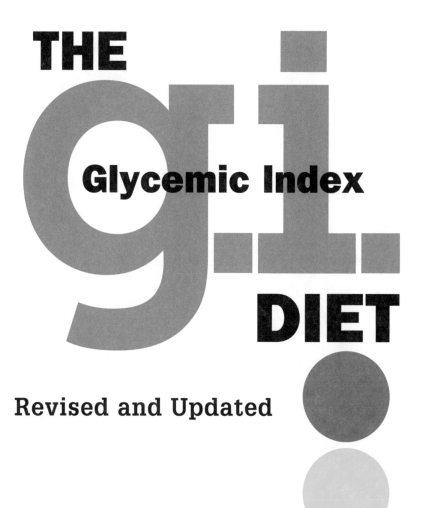

THE g.i. DIET

Glycemic Index

Revised and Updated

RICK GALLOP

FOREWORD BY Michael J. Sole, MD

workman publishing ▪ new york

First published in somewhat different form by
Random House Canada.

This U.S. edition published by arrangement with
Random House Canada, a division of Random House
of Canada Limited.

Library of Congress Cataloging-in-Publication Data
is available.

ISBN 978-0-7611-4479-3

Workman books are available at special discounts
when purchased in bulk for premiums and sales
promotions as well as for fund-raising or educational
use. Special editions or book excerpts can also be
created to specification. For details, contact the
Special Sales Director at the address below.

Workman Publishing Company, Inc.
225 Varick Street
New York, NY 10014-4381

www.workman.com

Printed in the United States of America
First printing December 2009

10 9 8 7 6 5 4 3 2 1

Acknowledgments

While I was writing the original *G.I. Diet,* I was also running the Heart and Stroke Foundation of Ontario, which had thirty-six offices and forty-five thousand volunteers and raised more than $100 million annually. The book was an enormous drain on my family time, and my wife, Ruth, bore the brunt of my preoccupation. Despite this, she was my cheerleader, culinary adviser, and coach. Without her encouragement and support, I doubt that I would have ever completed this book.

Dr. Michael Sole, cardiologist and researcher, provided invaluable advice and counsel. I am also deeply indebted to the late Dr. Ed Sonnenblick, who was one of the most eminent cardiologists in the United States, for believing in the value of the G.I. Diet and writing the foreword to the first editon of this book.

Among the many sources of information on the glycemic index, the most authoritative voice is Professor Jennie Brand-Miller at the University of Sydney. Her pioneering work in this field has been truly outstanding.

My thanks to my friends at Random House of Canada and Workman Publishing in New York: Anne Collins for encouraging me to write the book and Stacey Cameron, Suzanne Rafer, Beth Doty, and more recently, Erin Klabunde, for keeping me on track with wonderful editing and direction.

Finally, I must thank all my friends and associates who took part in my dietary research. Their feedback provided the focus and essence of the G.I. Diet.

Contents

Foreword

It's hard to ignore, especially as a cardiologist, the fact that obesity has ballooned into a crisis of epidemic proportions in North America. It affects one in three adults and one in four children and teenagers. In my own practice, I see a disproportionate number of patients who are overweight or obese, because obesity is a recognized risk factor for conditions that lay the foundation for heart attack and stroke. Millions of people are on diets, spending billions of dollars on self-help, quick-fix books; weight-loss programs; diet drinks; and foods. Obesity is a chronic condition, and effective weight management requires a long-term behavioral strategy. Many diets offer false promises of quick and easy weight loss, but these programs will not result in long-term success. The marked early weight loss seen in low-carbohydrate diets, for example, is due to water loss with depletion of carbohydrate (glycogen) stores, not fat loss. These diets are high in protein and fat and low in fiber and several important micronutrients; thus, they provide no basis for long-term healthful eating and permanent maintenance of weight loss. These diets also are associated with an increase in constipation and headache, and there is concern in the medical community that they pose an increased risk of cardiovascular disease and cancer.

Why read *The G.I. Diet,* another on a long shelf of "New You" promises? If you want weight-loss fiction, this book isn't for you. *The G.I. Diet* is an innovative, realistic, uncomplicated, long-term approach to successful weight management. To create this diet, Rick Gallop has drawn on his long experience with the Heart and Stroke Foundation of Ontario and its research and public education programs. He discusses the principles of nutrition and illustrates these with anecdotes and humor.

Building on this practical knowledge, Rick then tackles the challenge of weight loss as a long-term issue. He discusses a plan for changing unhealthy behaviors surrounding food, as well as the development of specific, achievable goals. *The G.I. Diet* presents the reader with a simple guide to food choices, both at home and away, with easy-to-remember images, practical tips, tasty recipes, and strategies for feedback and self-monitoring. Rick has also included an assortment of weight-loss tools—additions that the reader is certain to find useful. You only live once, and food is one of life's great pleasures. No one wants to spend time counting calories.

With a heavy travel schedule, lunchtime meetings, and dinners out, I must be continually vigilant about my weight. The principles and ideas described by Rick in this book have certainly been beneficial to me. *The G.I. Diet* charts a course that, if followed, will deliver on its promise of permanent weight loss.

—Michael J. Sole, BSC (Hon), MD,
FRCP(C), FACC, FAHA, FCAHS

Fellow of the American College of Cardiology and the American Heart Association
Former Chief of Cardiology, University Health Network
Professor of Medicine and Physiology
Founder of The Heart and Stroke/Richard Lewar Centre of Excellence,
University of Toronto

Introduction

I am so amazed and delighted by the number of people who have picked up *The G.I. Diet,* followed its advice, and slimmed down to their ideal weight. In a world of fad diets and bad advice, hundreds of thousands of people have chosen the best and healthiest way to permanent weight loss—hooray! The book has become a national bestseller in the United States, Canada, and Britain, and is now available in more than twenty countries in seventeen languages. And every day, I receive readers' letters and e-mails telling me how much weight they've lost and how it's changed their lives. This truly has been my greatest reward and satisfaction, because this is exactly what I set out to do when I first wrote the book: to help people get healthy and feel good about themselves.

I know what it's like to be overweight and to try one deprivation diet after another with no success. Several years ago, as a result of a lower-back disc problem, I had to give up my regular morning jog. Well, it didn't take long for me to gain 22 pounds and—even worse for my vanity—4 inches on my waist. As president of the Heart and Stroke Foundation of Ontario, my job was to raise funds for research into heart disease and stroke and to promote healthy lifestyle choices to reduce people's risk for those diseases. And there I was, overweight myself! All of a sudden I had to practice what I had been preaching for ten years—a sobering experience. I tried about a dozen different leading diets, but failed miserably every time. These diets presented three major roadblocks that frustrated my efforts to lose weight.

First, I was always hungry or feeling deprived. Second, these diets required counting calories, points, or carbs, which was far too time-consuming and complex for my busy schedule. Finally, I felt lethargic—lacking energy and just not feeling good.

Luckily, when I was just about at the end of my rope, I happened upon a way of eating that changed my life. I finally lost the weight that had been plaguing me for so long, and it was a revelation. You can imagine how excited I was; I wanted to tell everyone about it and end their dieting frustrations forever.

The result was *The G.I. Diet,* and the question of whether it works has been answered by the tens of thousands of e-mails I've received. Readers told me that they were losing weight without feeling hungry or deprived. They loved not having to count calories or points and were finding new energy levels that they hadn't experienced since their youth.

Included in this overwhelming reader response were questions and suggestions about how the G.I. Diet could be further refined to meet various lifestyle or health needs. This encouraged me to undertake additional research, which resulted in a series of G.I. Diet books targeted at meeting these needs. For example, I wrote *Living the G.I. Diet* for those who wanted more green-light recipes and, more recently, *The G.I. Diet Clinic,* a book based on an actual e-Clinic I conducted for people with significant weight problems.

Having accumulated a great deal of new knowledge from the preparation of these books, I decided it was time to revise and update the original *G.I. Diet.* This book includes new foods added to the red-, yellow-, and green-light food listings, as well as updates on maintaining good health; supplements; and exercise. I have also added new chapters or sections on eating out (at both family-style and fast-food restaurants), changing behaviors, emotional eating, staying motivated, falling off the wagon, and overcoming a weight-loss plateau—all this, plus a host of personal stories to help motivate you with your own weight-loss goals. I look forward to receiving your comments and suggestions through my website, www.gidiet.com.

The greatest dream in life is to feel you have made a difference to someone. I'd like to express my appreciation to those hundreds of thousands of readers who have made this dream come true for me!

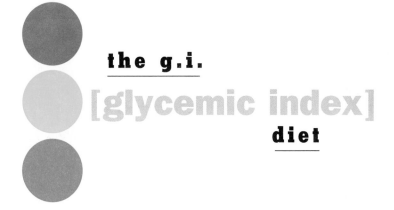

the g.i.
[glycemic index]
diet

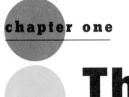
The
Problem

While I was waging my personal battle of the bulge, I couldn't help but be struck by the number of people who were engaged in the same struggle. The statistics are truly astonishing: 66 percent of American adults are overweight and an incredible one in three—more than double the rate of twenty years ago—is obese. The United States unfortunately leads the international stage in the heavyweight stakes.

What's happened to us? Why have we gained so much weight in the past twenty years?

The simple explanation is that people are eating too many calories. Unless one denies the basic laws of thermodynamics, the equation never changes: Consume more calories than you expend and the surplus is stored in the body as fat. That's the inescapable fact. But that doesn't explain why people today are eating more calories than they used to. To answer that question, we must first understand the three key components of any diet—fats, carbohydrates, and proteins—and how they function in our digestive system. Since fats are probably the least well understood, let's start with them.

FATS

Fat is definitely a bad word these days, and it engenders an enormous amount of confusion and contradiction. But are you aware that fats are absolutely essential to your diet? They contain several key elements that are crucial to the digestive process.

The next fact might also surprise you: Fat does not necessarily make you fat. The quantity you consume does. And that's something that's often difficult to control, because your body *loves* fat. Nonfat foods require lots of processing to be transformed into those fat cells around your waist and hips; fatty foods just slide right in. Processing takes energy, and your body hates wasting energy. It needs to expend about 20 to 25 percent of the energy it gets from a nonfat food just to process it. So your body definitely prefers fat, and as we all know from personal experience, it will do everything it can to persuade you to eat more of it. That's why fatty foods like juicy steaks, chocolate cake, and decadent ice cream taste so good to us. But because fat contains twice as many calories per gram as carbohydrates and proteins, we really have to be careful about the amount of fat we eat.

In addition to limiting *how much* fat we consume, we must also pay attention to the *type* of fat. While the type of fat has no effect on our weight, it is critical to our health—especially our heart health.

There are four types of fat: the best, the better, the bad, and the really ugly.

The "really ugly" fats are potentially the most dangerous. They are vegetable oils that have been heat-treated to make them thicken. These hydrogenated oils, or trans-fatty acids, take on the worst characteristics of saturated fats (see below), so don't use them, and avoid snack foods, baked goods, and cereals that contain them. Check the label for "hydrogenated oils," "partially hydrogenated oils," or "trans fat."

The "bad" fats are called saturated fats, and they are easily recognizable because they almost always come from animal

COOKING OILS/FATS

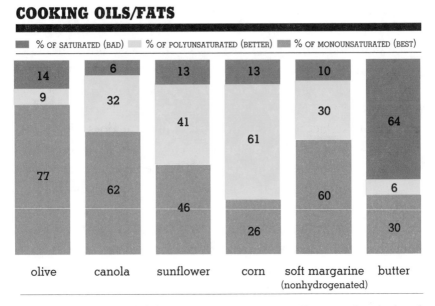

■ % OF SATURATED (BAD)　■ % OF POLYUNSATURATED (BETTER)　■ % OF MONOUNSATURATED (BEST)

olive	canola	sunflower	corn	soft margarine (nonhydrogenated)	butter
14	6	13	13	10	—
9	32	41	61	30	64
77	62	46	26	60	6 / 30

sources and they solidify at room temperature. Butter, cheese, hard (stick) margarine, and meat are all high in saturated fats. There are a couple of others you should be aware of, too. Coconut oil and palm oil are two vegetable oils that are saturated, and because they are cheap, they are used in many snack foods, especially cookies. Saturated fats are a principal cause of heart disease because they boost cholesterol, which in turn thickens arteries and causes heart attack and stroke. And recent research has demonstrated that several cancers (breast, colon, and prostate) as well as Alzheimer's disease are associated with diets high in saturated fat.

The "better" fats are called polyunsaturated fats, and they are cholesterol-free. Most vegetable oils, such as corn and sunflower, fall into this category.

What you should really be eating, however, are monounsaturated fats, the "best," which are found in olives, peanuts, almonds, and olive and canola oils. Monounsaturated fats have a beneficial effect on cholesterol and are good for your heart. (See chapter 11, Health, for more information on cholesterol and heart disease.) Though fancy olive oils are expensive, you can get the same health benefits from reasonably priced house brands at your supermarket. Olive oil is used extensively in the famed Mediterranean diet, which is also rich in fruits and vegetables. Because of their diet, southern Europeans have some of the lowest rates of heart disease in the world, and obesity is not a problem in those countries. So look for monounsaturated fats and oils on food labels. Most manufacturers who use them will say so, because they know it's a key selling point for informed consumers.

Another highly beneficial oil, which is in a category of its own, contains a wonderful ingredient called omega-3, found in deep-sea fish such as salmon and in flaxseed and canola oils. It's extremely good for your heart health (see page 137).

So we know that it's important to avoid the bad and the really ugly fats and to incorporate the best fats into our diets to make our hearts healthy. Many of us have tried to lower our fat intake by using leaner cuts of meat and drinking lower-fat milk. But even with these modifications, our fat consumption hasn't decreased. Why? Because many of our favorite foods—such as crackers, muffins, cereals, and fast foods—contain hidden fats. Detecting them often seems to require an advanced degree in nutrition, even with the labeling of nutritional components on food packaging.

So we're not eating less fat, but contrary to popular belief, neither are we eating more. Fat consumption in this country has remained virtually constant over the past ten years, while overweight numbers have doubled. Obviously, fat isn't the culprit. What *has* increased is our consumption of grain. Grain is a carbohydrate, so let's look at how carbohydrates work.

---

to sum up

1. Eat less fat overall, and look for low-fat alternatives to incorporate into your current diet.

2. Eat monounsaturated and polyunsaturated fats only.

CARBOHYDRATES

Unfortunately, there is a great deal of misinformation in the marketplace about carbohydrates. Much of it stems from the recent low-carb diet fad, which would have you believe that if you stick to eating low-carb foods, you'll lose weight. If only it were that simple. The reality is that you need carbs for a healthy diet, and you shouldn't avoid them. The key is to choose the right, or good, carbs, like fruits, vegetables, legumes, whole grains, nuts, and low-fat dairy products. These foods are the primary sources of energy for your body, which converts them into glucose. The glucose dissolves in your bloodstream and is diverted to those parts of the body that use energy, like your muscles and your brain. (It may surprise you to know that when you are resting, your brain uses about two thirds of the glucose in your system!)

Carbohydrates, therefore, are essential for your body to function. They are rich in fiber, vitamins, and minerals, including antioxidants, which we now believe play a critical role in protecting against disease, especially heart disease and cancer. For years we've been advised by doctors, nutritionists, and the government to eat a low-fat, high-carbohydrate diet, and this trend is reflected in our supermarkets. Just look at the amount of space dedicated to carbohydrates in our grocery stores: huge cracker, cookie, and snack-food sections; whole aisles of cereals; numerous shelves of pastas and noodles; and baskets and baskets of bagels, rolls, muffins, and loaves of bread. Most food stores carry half a dozen different bagel varieties, and chains of bagel, doughnut, and cookie stores are spread across the country. Muffins were never as abundant as they are today.

Another modern food sensation is pasta, once viewed as an ethnic specialty in the United States and Canada. That's hard to believe today, with pasta as a staple on most restaurant menus and every family's shopping list. U.S. pasta consumption has nearly doubled over the past ten years or so. And our snack-food options

GRAIN CONSUMPTION (POUNDS PER CAPITA)

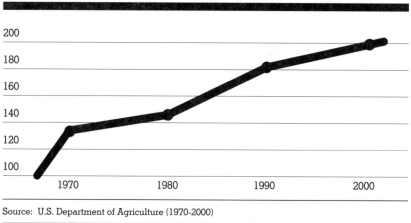

Source: U.S. Department of Agriculture (1970-2000)

have multiplied: crackers, tortilla chips, potato chips, and pretzels, to name just a few.

In 1970, the average American ate about 135 pounds of grain per year. By 2000, that figure had risen to *200* pounds. That's nearly a 50 percent increase! But why should we be concerned about this? Aren't wheat, corn, and rice low-fat? How could grain be making us fat?

The answer lies in the *type* of grain we're eating today, most of which is in the form of white flour. White flour starts off as whole wheat. At the mill, the whole wheat is steamed and scarified by tiny razor-sharp blades to remove the bran, or outer shell, and the endosperm, the next layer. Then the wheat germ and oil are removed because they turn rancid too quickly to be considered commercially viable. What's left after all that processing is unbleached flour, which is then whitened and used to make almost all the breads, bagels, muffins, cookies, crackers, cereals, and pastas we consume. Even many "brown" breads are simply artificially colored white bread.

It's not just grain that's highly processed nowadays. A hundred years ago, most of the food people ate came straight from the farm to the dinner table. Lack of refrigeration and scant knowledge of food chemistry meant that most food remained in its original state. However, advances in science, along with the migration of many women out of the kitchen and into the workforce, led to a revolution in prepared foods. Everything became geared to speed and simplicity of preparation. Today's high-speed flour mills use steel rollers rather than the traditional grinding stones to produce an extraordinarily fine-ground product, ideal for producing light and fluffy breads and pastries. We now have instant rice and potatoes, as well as entire meals that are ready to eat after just a few minutes in the microwave.

The trouble with all this is that the more a food is processed beyond its natural state, the less processing your body has to do to digest it. And the quicker you digest your food, the sooner you're hungry again and the more you tend to eat. We all know the difference between eating a bowl of old-fashioned slow-cooked oatmeal and a bowl of sugary cold cereal. The oatmeal stays with you—it "sticks to your ribs," as my mother used to say—whereas you're looking for your next meal an hour after eating the bowl of sugary cereal. That's why our ancestors did not have the obesity problem we have today; their foods were basically unprocessed and natural. All of the major food companies, such as Kraft, Kellogg's, McCain, Nabisco, and Del Monte, only started processing and packaging natural foods in the past century.

Our fundamental problem, then, is that we're eating foods that are too easily digested by our bodies. Clearly, we can't wind back the clock to simpler times, but we need somehow to slow down the digestive process so we feel hungry less often. How can we do that? Well, we have to eat foods that are "slow release," that break down at a slow and steady rate in our digestive system, leaving us feeling fuller for longer periods of time.

The principal tool in identifying slow-release foods is the Glycemic Index, which I will now explain. It is the core of this diet and the key to successful weight management.

THE GLYCEMIC INDEX

The Glycemic Index measures the speed at which you digest food and convert it to glucose, your body's energy source. The faster the food breaks down, the higher the rating on the index. The index sets sugar (glucose) at 100 and scores all foods against that number. Here are some examples:

GLYCEMIC INDEX RATINGS

sugar (glucose) = 100

Baguette	95	Orange	44
Rice (instant)	87	All-Bran	43
Cornflakes	84	Oatmeal	42
Potato (baked)	84	Peach	42
Doughnut	76	Spaghetti	41
Cheerios	75	Tomato	38
Bagel	72	Apple	38
Raisins	64	Yogurt (low-fat)	33
Rice (basmati)	58	Fettuccine	32
Muffin (bran)	56	Beans	31
Potato (new/boiled)	56	Grapefruit	25
Popcorn (microwave light)	55	Yogurt (fat-free with sweetener)	14

The chart on page 10 illustrates the impact of sugar on the level of glucose in your bloodstream compared with kidney beans, which have a low G.I. rating. As you can see, there is a dramatic difference between the two. Sugar is quickly converted into glucose, which dissolves in your bloodstream, spiking the blood's glucose level. Sugars also disappear quickly, leaving you wanting more. Have you ever eaten a large Chinese meal, with lots of noodles and rice, only to find yourself hungry again an hour or two later? That's because your body rapidly converted the rice and noodles, both high-G.I. foods, to glucose, which then quickly disappeared from your bloodstream. Something most of us experience regularly is the lethargy that follows an hour or so after a fast-food lunch, which generally consists of high-G.I. foods. The surge of glucose followed by the rapid drain leaves us starved of energy. So what do we do? Around midafternoon, we look for a quick sugar fix to bring us out of the slump. A few cookies or a bag of chips causes another rush of glucose, which disappears a short time later—and so the vicious cycle continues. No wonder we're a nation of snackers!

When you eat a high-G.I. food and experience a rapid spike in blood sugar, your pancreas releases the hormone insulin. Insulin does two things extremely well. First, it reduces the level of glucose in your bloodstream by diverting it into various body tissues for immediate short-term use or by storing it as fat—which is why glucose disappears so quickly. Second, it inhibits the conversion of body fat back into glucose for the body to burn. This evolutionary feature is a throwback to the days when our ancestors were hunter-gatherers, habitually experiencing times of feast or famine. When food was in abundance, the body stored its surplus as fat to tide it over during the inevitable days of famine. Insulin was the champion in this process, both helping to accumulate fat and then guarding against its depletion.

G.I. IMPACT ON SUGAR LEVELS

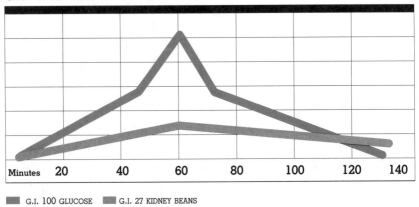

| Minutes | 20 | 40 | 60 | 80 | 100 | 120 | 140 |

G.I. 100 GLUCOSE   G.I. 27 KIDNEY BEANS

Today, everything has changed except our stomachs. A digestive system that has taken millions of years to evolve is, in a comparative blink of an eye, expected to cope with a food revolution. We don't have to hunt for food anymore; we have a guaranteed supply of highly processed foods with a multitude of tempting flavors and textures at the supermarket. Not only are we consuming more easily digested calories, but we're not expending as much energy in finding our food and keeping ourselves warm— the two major preoccupations of our ancestors.

Since insulin is the key trigger to storing glucose, as well as the sentry that keeps those fat cells intact, it is crucial to maintain low insulin levels when you are trying to lose weight, and that means avoiding high-G.I. foods. Low-G.I. foods, such as apples, are like the tortoise to the high-G.I. foods' hare. They break down in your digestive system at a slow, steady rate. You don't get a quick sugar fix when you eat them, but tortoiselike, they stay the course, so you feel full longer. Therefore, if you want to lose weight, you must stick to low-G.I. foods.

But the fact that a food has a low G.I. rating does not necessarily make it desirable. The other critical factor in determining whether a food will allow you to lose weight is its calorie content. It's the combination of low-G.I. foods with few calories—that is, low in sugar and/or fat—that is the "magic bullet" of the G.I. Diet. Low-G.I., low-calorie foods make you feel more satiated than do foods with a high G.I. and calorie level. Later in this book, I will provide a comprehensive chart identifying the foods that will make you gain weight and those that will allow you to lose it. Don't expect low-G.I. foods to be tasteless and boring! There are many delicious and satisfying choices that will make you feel as though you aren't even on a diet.

There are three other important things that inhibit the rapid breakdown of a food in our digestive system, and they are fiber, fat, and protein.

Fiber, in simple terms, provides low-calorie filler. In fact, it does double duty. Fiber literally fills up your stomach, so you feel satiated; and your body takes much longer to break it down, so it stays with you longer and slows down the digestive process. There are two forms of fiber: soluble and insoluble. Soluble fiber is found in foods like oatmeal, beans, barley, and citrus fruits, and has been shown to lower blood cholesterol levels. Insoluble fiber is important for normal bowel function and is typically found in whole wheat breads and cereals, and in most vegetables.

Fat, like fiber, acts like a brake in the digestive process. When combined with other foods, it becomes a barrier to digestive juices. It also signals the brain that you are satisfied and do not require more food. But we know that many fats are harmful to your heart, and they contain twice the number of calories per gram as carbohydrates and protein. Since protein also acts as a brake in the digestive process, let's look at it in more detail.

PROTEIN

One half of your dry body weight is made up of protein, i.e., your muscles, internal organs, skin, and hair. Obviously, protein is an essential part of your diet. It's required to build and repair body tissue, and it figures in nearly all metabolic reactions.

Protein is also much more effective than carbohydrates or fat in satisfying hunger. It will make you feel fuller longer, which is why you should always try to incorporate some protein into every meal and snack. It will also help keep you alert. Again, however, the type of protein you consume is important. Proteins are found in a broad range of food products, both animal and vegetable, and not just in red meat and whole dairy products, which are high in saturated, or "bad," fats.

So what sort of protein should you include in your diet? Choose low-fat proteins: lean or low-fat meats that have been trimmed of any visible fat; skinless poultry; fresh, frozen, or canned seafood (but not the kind that's coated with batter, which is invariably high in fat); low-fat dairy products such as skim milk (believe it or not, after a couple of weeks of drinking it, it tastes just like 2%); low-fat yogurt (look for the artificially sweetened versions, as many manufacturers pump up the sugar as they drop the fat) and low-fat cottage cheese; low-cholesterol liquid eggs or egg whites; and tofu. To most people's surprise, the best source of protein may well be the humble bean. Beans are high-protein, low-fat, and high-fiber, and they break down slowly in your digestive system, keeping you full. They can also be added to foods like soups and salads to boost their protein and fiber content. Nuts, too, are a fine source of protein, with a good monounsaturated fat content. However, because they are so high in calories, you must limit the quantity you consume.

One of the most important things you should know about protein is to spread your daily allowance across all your meals. Too often we grab a hasty breakfast of coffee and toast—a protein-free meal. Lunch is sometimes not much better: a bowl of hot vegetable soup or a green salad with garlic bread. Where's the protein? A typical afternoon snack of a cookie, a piece of fruit, or chips contains not a gram of protein. Generally, it's not until dinner that we include protein in our meal, usually our entire daily recommended allowance, plus some extra. Because protein is a critical brain food, providing amino acids for the neurotransmitters that relay messages in the brain, it would be better to load up on protein earlier in the day rather than later. That would give you an alert and active mind for your daily activities. However, as I have said, the best solution is to spread your protein consumption throughout the day. This will help keep you on the ball and feeling full.

Now that we know how fats, carbohydrates, and proteins work in our digestive system and what makes us gain weight, let's use the science to put together an eating plan that will take off the extra pounds. First, though, let's look at how much weight you should be trying to lose.

to sum up

1. Low-G.I. foods are slower to digest, so you feel satiated longer.

2. Keeping insulin levels low inhibits the formation of fat and assists in the conversion of fat back into energy.

3. The key to losing weight is to eat low-G.I., low-calorie foods.

chapter two

How Much Weight Should I Lose?

In this age of excessively and often unhealthily skinny super-models and TV stars, it's easy to lose sight of what is a healthy weight. Your skin, bones, internal organs, and hair all contribute to your body's total weight. The only part that you want to reduce is your excess fat, so that's what we have to determine.

There have been many techniques designed to measure excess fat, from measuring pinches of fat (which can be quite misleading) to convoluted formulas and tables requiring higher math. The traditional method, relating weight directly to height through the Metropolitan Life tables, does not tell you how much body fat you're carrying around your waist, hips, and thighs, and that's the information you really need to know. So the best method is the Body Mass Index, or BMI. I've included a BMI table on pages 16–17, and it's very simple to use. Just find your height in the left vertical column and go across the table until you reach your weight. At the top of that column is your BMI, which is an accurate estimate of the amount of body fat you're carrying.

BODY MASS INDEX (BMI)

	normal						overweight					obese		
BMI	19	20	21	22	23	24	25	26	27	28	29	30	31	32
height (inches)	body weight (pounds)													
4'10"	91	96	100	105	110	115	119	124	129	134	138	143	148	153
4'11"	94	99	104	109	114	119	124	128	133	138	143	148	153	158
5'0"	97	102	107	112	118	123	128	133	138	143	148	153	158	163
5'1"	100	106	111	116	122	127	132	137	143	148	153	158	164	169
5'2"	104	109	115	120	126	131	136	142	147	153	158	164	169	175
5'3"	107	113	118	124	130	135	141	146	152	158	163	169	175	180
5'4"	110	116	122	128	134	140	145	151	157	163	169	174	180	186
5'5"	114	120	126	132	138	144	150	156	162	168	174	180	186	192
5'6"	118	124	130	136	142	148	155	161	167	173	179	186	192	198
5'7"	121	127	134	140	146	153	159	166	172	178	185	191	198	204
5'8"	125	131	138	144	151	158	164	171	177	184	190	197	203	210
5'9"	128	135	142	149	155	162	169	176	182	189	196	203	209	216
5'10"	132	139	146	153	160	167	174	181	188	195	202	209	216	222
5'11"	136	143	150	157	165	172	179	186	193	200	208	215	222	229
6'0"	140	147	154	162	169	177	184	191	199	206	213	221	228	235
6'1"	144	151	159	166	174	182	189	197	204	212	219	227	235	242
6'2"	148	155	163	171	179	186	194	202	210	218	225	233	241	249
6'3"	152	160	168	176	184	192	200	208	216	224	232	240	248	256
6'4"	156	164	172	180	189	197	205	213	221	230	238	246	254	263

Source: U.S. National Heart, Lung, and Blood Institute

extreme obesity

33	34	(35)	36	37	38	39	40	41	42	43	44	45	46	47	48	49
158	162	167	172	177	181	186	191	196	201	205	210	215	220	224	229	234
163	168	173	178	183	188	193	198	203	208	212	217	222	227	232	237	242
168	174	179	184	189	194	199	204	209	215	220	225	230	235	240	245	250
174	180	185	190	195	201	206	211	217	222	227	232	238	243	248	254	259
180	186	191	196	202	207	213	218	224	229	235	240	246	251	256	262	267
186	191	197	203	208	214	220	225	231	237	242	248	254	259	265	270	278
192	197	204	209	215	221	227	232	238	244	250	256	262	267	273	279	285
198	204	210	216	222	228	234	240	246	252	258	264	270	276	282	288	294
204	210	216	223	229	235	241	247	253	260	266	272	278	284	291	297	303
211	217	223	230	236	242	249	255	261	268	274	280	287	293	299	306	312
216	223	230	236	243	249	256	262	269	276	282	289	295	302	308	315	322
223	230	236	243	250	257	263	270	277	284	291	297	304	311	318	324	331
229	236	243	250	257	264	271	278	285	292	299	306	313	320	327	334	341
236	243	250	257	265	272	279	286	293	301	308	315	322	329	338	343	351
242	250	258	265	272	279	287	294	302	309	316	324	331	338	346	353	361
250	257	265	272	280	288	295	302	310	318	325	333	340	348	355	363	371
256	264	272	280	287	295	303	311	319	326	334	342	350	358	365	373	381
264	272	279	287	295	303	311	319	327	335	343	351	359	367	375	383	391
271	279	287	295	304	312	320	328	336	344	353	361	369	377	385	394	402

BMI tables have a broad range of weights in each of the weight categories: healthy weight (BMI 19 to 24), overweight (BMI 25 to 29), and obese (BMI 30 and over). For instance, a woman who is 5 feet 5 inches tall has a healthy weight range of 114 pounds (BMI 19) to 144 pounds (BMI 24). The reason for this broad range is primarily to allow for variances in the size of people's frames.

Women with small frames should have a healthy weight that falls in the bottom third of the range, while those with large frames should fall in the top third. For example, a woman with a small frame should have a BMI of 19 to 21; medium frame, BMI 21 to 22; large frame, BMI 23 to 24.

To calculate which size frame you fit into, use this guide based on your wrist size. Wrap a tape measure around the narrowest point on your wrist.

DETERMINING MEN'S AND WOMEN'S FRAME SIZES

| WOMAN'S WRIST | HEIGHT | | |
SIZE (INCHES)	UNDER 5'2"	5'2"–5'5"	OVER 5'5"
Under 5.50	S	S	S
5.50–5.75	M	S	S
5.75–6.00	L	S	S
6.00–6.25	L	M	S
6.25–6.50	L	L	M
Over 6.50	L	L	L

Key: S = small frame; M = medium frame; L = large frame

FOR A MALE IT IS A LITTLE SIMPLER:

Under 6.5 inches =	small frame
6.5–7.5 inches =	medium frame
Over 7.5 inches =	large frame

Source: U.S. National Library of Medicine

If you're over 65 years old, I suggest you allow yourself an extra 10 pounds to help protect you in case of a fall or long illness. Basically, everyone has his or her own particular body makeup, metabolism, and genes, so there are no hard-and-fast rules for exactly how much you should weigh. The BMI table is a guide, not an absolute. However, it is important that *you* set your goals and write them down. Everyone has different motivations for losing weight, and neither I nor the BMI tables can do this for you.

Remember, you are starting on a journey. Don't expect miracles. The weight will come off. For those with a BMI of over 30 who may feel overwhelmed by the task ahead, you do have one advantage over your skinnier compatriots in that you will lose weight at a faster rate.

Say you've decided to target a BMI of 22. Turn to the table on page 16. Put your finger on the BMI number 22 and drop down until you reach your height, which is shown in the left margin. The number at that intersection is what your weight should be when you achieve your BMI target. Let's look at an example: Mary is 5 feet 6 inches tall with a medium frame and weighs 180 pounds. Her current BMI is 29, but she'd like to have a BMI of 22. This means Mary has to lose 44 pounds in order to bring her to her 22 BMI goal of 136 pounds.

Another measurement that is important to know is your waist circumference. This measurement is an even better indication of your health than your weight is. Recent research has shown that abdominal fat acts almost like a separate organ in the body—only this "organ" is a destructive one. It releases harmful proteins and free fatty acids, increasing the risk of heart disease, stroke, cancer, and diabetes. Thus, women with a waist circumference of 35 inches or more and men whose waists measure 37 inches or more are at risk of endangering their health. And women with a waist circumference of 37 inches or more and men with 40 inches or more are at serious risk of heart disease, stroke, cancer, and diabetes. Doctors often describe people with abdominal fat as apple-shaped.

To determine your waist size, wrap a measuring tape around your natural waist just above the navel. Don't be tempted to do a walk-down-the-beach-sucking-it-in routine. Just stand in a relaxed position and keep the measuring tape from cutting into your flesh.

The 44 pounds that Mary has to lose are pounds of fat—Mary's energy storage tank. In order for her to lose weight, she must access and draw down those fat cells. This reminds me of a peculiar contraption used in England during World War II. The famous double-decker buses were converted to run on natural gas and had their upper deck changed into a natural gas tank consisting of a large fabric balloon. When full, the balloon puffed up several feet above the top of the bus. As it proceeded along its route, the balloon slowly deflated, disappearing by the time the bus reached its destination, where it was reinflated. That's how I visualize our body fat: a deflating balloon from which we draw down our energy, except that in our case the balloon is around our waist, hips, and thighs.

So how do you draw down energy from your fat cells? By consuming fewer calories than your body needs. This will force your body to start using its fat stores to make up for the shortfall. Now, I know no one wants to hear about calories, particularly those of us who've tried long and hard to lose weight. Nevertheless, unless you are among those rare and blessed people whose metabolism and genetics enable them to eat as much as they want without gaining an ounce—and if you are, why would you be reading this book?—you, like me and the rest of us mere mortals, are doomed to the inevitable equation. But don't be disheartened. You can easily reduce your daily calorie intake without going hungry and without having to calculate the number of calories in everything you put into your mouth.

I promised you a simple eating plan that reflects the real world we live in, and that is what I'll give you. The plan is divided into two phases. In Phase I, you'll be reducing your caloric intake, burning off those excess fat cells, and slimming down to a healthy, ideal weight.

For most people it's really a matter of simple math. A pound of fat contains around 3,600 calories. To lose that pound in one week, you must reduce your caloric intake by around 500 calories per day (500 × 7 days = 3,500 calories). So if you want to lose 20 pounds, it will take 20 weeks. But this formula is for people who have to lose about 10 percent of their body weight. If you have more to lose, the good news is that you will in all likelihood drop more pounds per week. The higher your BMI, the faster you will lose weight. People with a BMI of 30 or higher frequently lose an average of 2 to 3 pounds per week.

If twenty weeks seems like a long time to you, think of it in terms of the rest of your life. What's half a year compared with the many, many years you'll spend afterward with a slim, healthy body? This isn't a fad diet—fad diets don't work. In fact, the sole reason that 95 percent of diets don't lead to permanent weight loss is simply that people can't or won't stay on them. And the reasons are very simple: People feel hungry or deprived; they get tired of counting calories, points, and carbs; and they feel lethargic and depressed.

With the G.I. Diet, however, you will not feel hungry or deprived; you'll never have to count calories again; and you will rediscover energy levels you thought you had lost forever. *The most important single message I can leave with you is that if you wish to permanently lose weight, then you have to permanently change the way you eat. The most common theme I hear from successful G.I. Diet readers is that this is not so much a diet as it is a new and permanent way of eating.* The G.I. Diet is a wholesome and surefire route to permanent weight loss.

I've included some math to help you understand this diet and how it's going to work for you. But I don't want you to think that you're going to have to do any calculations yourself! They're all built into the program. I've done all the math, calculations, and measurements for you, and sorted the foods you're likely to want to eat into one of three categories based on the colors of the traffic light. The easy-to-follow color-coded system means you will never have to count calories or points again.

And speaking of measurements, it is important that you calculate your weight accurately. Many of you are probably using scales you've had around for years, and chances are they're the analog type with a dial. Over time, springs stretch and they become wildly inaccurate. Do yourself a favor and purchase a digital scale. They can be bought for under $50.

PHASE II

When you've reached your target BMI, Phase II begins. Here, your caloric input and output are balanced. You're no longer trying to lose weight, so we relax the rules a little and you can start eating foods from the yellow-light category from time to time. All you're doing at this point is maintaining your new weight. This is how you'll be eating for the rest of your life. Sound simple? It is! So let's get going with Phase I.

---

to sum up

1. Set a realistic weight-loss target. A BMI of 19 to 24 should be your goal.

2. In Phase I of the G.I. Diet, you'll be reducing the number of calories you consume by eating low-G.I., low-calorie foods.

3. When you reach your target BMI, you'll start Phase II of the G.I. Diet, which evens out the number of calories you consume and expend.

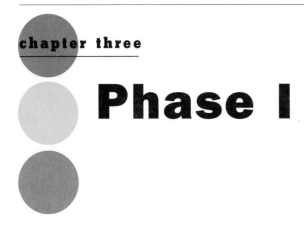

Phase I

With the theory and science of the G.I. Diet behind us, it's time to get practical! So let's get into the details of Phase I: what to eat, how much, and how often. This chapter summarizes the foods to eat and the foods to avoid. For a more complete list, check out the Complete G.I. Diet Food Guide on page 138. Here's how the color-coded categories work:

RED-LIGHT FOODS

The foods in the red column are to be avoided. They are high-G.I., higher-calorie foods and frequently have high saturated fat levels. Your body digests these foods so quickly that they're just not worth it.

YELLOW-LIGHT FOODS

The foods in the yellow column are midrange G.I. foods and should be treated with caution. During Phase I, the weight-loss portion of the diet, yellow-light foods should be avoided. Once you've reached your target weight and have entered Phase II—the maintenance phase—you can begin to enjoy yellow-light foods.

GREEN-LIGHT FOODS

The green column lists foods that are low-G.I., low in saturated fat, and lower in calories. These are the foods that will help you lose weight. There's a green-light food for every craving, and the wide variety of tasty choices will ensure that you never feel deprived. You might be surprised to find potatoes and rice in the green-light column—they're fine as long as they are the right type. Baked potatoes and French fries have a high G.I., while boiled small (preferably new) potatoes have a lower G.I. With rice, the short-grain, glutinous (sticky) variety served in Chinese and Thai restaurants is high G.I., while long-grain, brown, basmati, and wild are low. Pasta is also a green-light food—as long as it is cooked al dente (with some firmness to the bite).

Any processing of food, including cooking, will raise its G.I., since heat breaks down food starch capsules and fiber, giving your digestive juices a head start. This is why you should never overcook vegetables; instead, microwave or steam them until they're tender. This way they will retain their vitamins and other nutrients and their G.I. rating will remain low. Remember, the objective is to digest foods slowly, and anything that increases the speed of digestion—such as raising the G.I. level of foods—is to be avoided. In this chapter, we will outline the best green-light options for breakfast, lunch, dinner, and snacks.

HOW MUCH DO I EAT?

The G.I. Diet calls for three meals and three snacks daily. As my mother liked to say, "The devil finds work for idle hands." Well, your stomach works on a similar principle in that if it's not kept busy processing food and steadily supplying energy to your brain and muscles, it will be looking for its next meal!

Portions

You can, with a few exceptions that I outline below (where specific portions or servings are indicated), eat as much of the green-light foods as you like. Specific portions are especially important in the case of foods that have a mid-range G.I. rating or are particularly

SPECIFIC PORTIONS

Crispbreads (with high fiber; e.g., Wasa Fiber)	2 crispbreads
Green-light breads (whole-grain, high-fiber; at least 3g fiber per slice)	1 slice
Green-light cereals	½ cup
Green-light nuts	8 to 10
Ice cream (low-fat, no added sugar)	½ cup
Soft margarine (nonhydrogenated, light)	2 teaspoons
Meat/seafood/poultry	4 ounces (about the size of a pack of cards)
Olive/canola oil	1 teaspoon
Olives	4 to 5
Pasta (whole wheat or protein-enriched)	¾ cup cooked
Potatoes (boiled small, preferably new)	2 to 3
Rice (basmati, brown, long-grain, wild)	⅔ cup cooked

Phase II

Chocolate (70% cocoa)	2 squares
Red wine	One 5-ounce glass

calorie-dense. This does, however, call for some common sense and moderation. Eating three oranges or two heads of cabbage at a sitting is not moderation! Each meal and snack should contain, if possible, a combination of green-light protein, carbohydrates—especially fruits and vegetables—and fats. An easy way to visualize portion size is to divide your plate into three sections (see the diagram on page 156). Half the plate should be filled with at least two vegetables; one quarter should contain protein, such as lean meat, poultry, seafood, tofu, liquid eggs or egg whites; and the last quarter should contain a green-light serving of rice, pasta, or potatoes.

One of the simplest ways to reduce your portion sizes is to change your huge dinner plates to luncheon-size plates. Research has shown that this is a highly effective way of reducing calorie intake without creating a feeling of being shortchanged.

WHEN DO I EAT?

Try to eat regularly throughout the day. If you skimp on breakfast and lunch, you'll probably be starving by dinner and end up over-eating. Have one snack midmorning, another midafternoon, and one before bed. The idea is to keep your digestive system happily busy so you won't start craving those red-light snacks.

PHASE I MEALS

So now that you know about food portions, what can you eat? Let's talk about breakfast first. The chart here lists breakfast foods in the three color-coded categories. Following the chart is an explanation of how certain popular foods are categorized. If a food is not included in the chart, it is usually because a rating has not yet been established.

For an extended list of the most popular food for all meals and snacks, see The Complete G.I. Diet Food Guide on page 138.

BREAKFAST

PROTEIN

	● RED LIGHT	● YELLOW LIGHT	● GREEN LIGHT
meat*/eggs	Bacon (regular) Sausages	Turkey bacon Whole eggs (preferably omega-3)	Canadian bacon Deli ham (lean) Egg Beaters Egg whites Liquid eggs
dairy	Cheese (regular) Cottage cheese (whole or 2%) Cream Cream cheese (regular) Milk (whole or 2%) Sour cream (regular) Yogurt (whole or 2%)	Cheese (low-fat) Cream cheese (light) Milk (1%) Sour cream (light) Yogurt (low-fat with sugar)	Buttermilk Cheese (fat-free) Cottage cheese (1% or fat-free) Cream cheese (nonfat) Extra-low-fat cheese Flavored yogurt (fat-free with sweetener) Milk (skim) Sour cream (1% or fat-free) Soy milk (plain, low-fat) Soy or whey protein powder

CARBOHYDRATES

	● RED LIGHT	● YELLOW LIGHT	● GREEN LIGHT
cereals	All cold cereals except those listed as yellow- or green-light	Post Shredded Wheat'N Bran	Homemade Muesli (see page 64)*

*Limit serving size (see page 25).

CARBOHYDRATES

	● RED LIGHT	● YELLOW LIGHT	● GREEN LIGHT
cereals (continued)	Cream of Wheat Granola Grits Instant/quick-cook oatmeal Muesli (commercial)		Cold cereals with at least 10g fiber or protein per serving (e.g., All-Bran, Bran Buds, Fiber One, Kashi GoLean, Kashi GoLean Crunch!)* Kasha* Kashi GoLean hot cereal* Large-flake, rolled, or steel-cut oats (e.g., Old-Fashioned Quaker Oats)* Oat bran*
breads/grains	Bagels Baguettes and other crusty white breads Croissants and pastries Doughnuts English muffins Granola bars (commercial) Muffins (commercial) Pancakes/waffles White bread	Crispbreads (with fiber; e.g., Ryvita High Fiber) Whole-grain breads (less than 3g fiber/slice)	Crispbreads (with high fiber; e.g., Wasa Fiber)* Homemade Apple Bran Muffins (see page 86) Homemade Granola Bars (see page 87) Whole-grain, high-fiber bread (at least 3g fiber per slice)*

*Limit serving size (see page 25).

	🔴 RED LIGHT	⚪ YELLOW LIGHT	⚫ GREEN LIGHT
fruits (fresh/ frozen/ dried/ canned)	Applesauce containing sugar Canned fruits in syrup (all) Cantaloupe Dried fruit (most)* Melons Raisins*	Apricots (dried)* Apricots (fresh) Bananas Cranberries (dried)* Fruit cocktail in juice Kiwis Mangoes Papayas Pineapple	Apples Applesauce (unsweetened) Berries Cherries Fruit spreads (double fruit, no added sugar) Grapefruit Grapes Oranges Peaches Pears Plums
juices	Fruit drinks (all) Prune Sweetened juices, including naturally sweetened (all) Watermelon	Apple (unsweetened) Cranberry (unsweetened) Grapefruit (unsweetened) Orange (unsweetened) Pear nectar (unsweetened) Pineapple (unsweetened)	Eat the fruit rather than drink its juice
vegetables**	French fries Hash browns/ home fries		Most vegetables

*You may use a modest amount of dried fruit for baking.

**See page 148 for complete list.

FATS

RED LIGHT	YELLOW LIGHT	GREEN LIGHT
Butter	Natural nut butters	Almonds*
Hard margarine		Canola oil*
Peanut butter (regular and light)	Natural peanut butter (100% peanuts)	Cashews*
		Hazelnuts*
	Nuts, except those listed as green-light	Macadamia nuts*
Tropical oils (such as palm and coconut)		Olive oil*
	Soft margarine (nonhydroge-nated)	Pistachios*
Vegetable shortening		Soft margarine (nonhyrdroge-nated, light; e.g., Promise Light)*
	Vegetable oils	

*Limit serving size (see page 25).

Juice/Fruit

- Always eat the fruit or vegetable rather than drink its juice. Juice is a processed product that is more rapidly digested than the parent fruit. To illustrate the point, diabetics who run into an insulin crisis and are in a state of hypoglycemia (low blood sugar) are usually given orange juice, which is the fastest way to get glucose into the bloodstream. A glass of juice has two and a half times the calories of a fresh whole orange. The "flesh" of the fruit also contains fiber and other nutrients, such as minerals, that aren't found in juice.

Cereals

- Large-flake or slow-cooking oats are the best choices for two reasons: Oatmeal stays with you all morning, and it's great for your heart because it lowers cholesterol. (The cooking time is only around three minutes in the microwave.) Oat bran is also an excellent choice.

- When choosing cold cereals, go for the high-fiber or high-protein products—the ones that have at least 10 grams of fiber or protein per serving. Fiber and protein content is clearly indicated on cereal packages. Cereal manufacturers, to their credit, were among the first to voluntarily publish nutritional facts.

- High-fiber cereals are a great base to which fruit, nuts, and yogurt may be added.

Dairy

- The beverage of choice is skim milk. I had a real problem with skim milk both on cereal and as a beverage, but I persevered. Move down from 2% to 1% to skim in stages. I find that 2% tastes like cream now!

- Yogurt is a real plus. But look for low-fat or nonfat versions with sugar substitute rather than sugar. Regular low-fat yogurts have nearly twice the calories as the versions with sweetener. (There has been a considerable amount of negative publicity, generated principally by the sugar industry, about sugar substitutes. This has triggered dozens of studies worldwide, none of which have shown that sugar substitutes pose any long-term risks to our health. These products are safe and of real value in calorie control. But as with most foods, don't go overboard.) Our family's favorite is Splenda, which, unlike aspartame, can also be used in baking.

- Cottage cheese is an excellent and filling source of protein. Again, go for the 1% or fat-free variety. Add fruit or light fruit spreads for flavor.

- Use other dairy products sparingly. Avoid most cheeses like the plague; their high saturated fat heads straight for your arteries. If cheese is your thing, then go for the nonfat options such as nonfat cream cheese, which is an excellent green-light product. Or use stronger-flavored ones, such as Stilton or feta, but only sprinkled sparingly as a flavor enhancer.

Bread

- Always use whole-grain, high-fiber bread that has a minimum of 3 grams of fiber per slice. Limit yourself to one slice per meal.

Eggs

- Use egg whites only, or low-cholesterol eggs in liquid form (a 250 ml carton = 5 eggs). Unlike regular eggs, which are high in cholesterol, liquid eggs are a great green-light product. Go for them.

Spreads/Preserves

- Do not use butter. The latest premium brands of nonhydrogenated soft margarine are acceptable and the light versions even more so, but use sparingly.

- Avoid all fruit spreads in which the first ingredient is sugar. Look for the "double fruit, no added sugar" versions. These taste terrific and are remarkably low in calories. They are wonderful flavor boosters for oatmeal, high-fiber cereal, and cottage cheese.

Bacon

- Sorry, but regular bacon is a red-light food. Acceptable alternatives are Canadian bacon and lean ham.

Coffee/Tea

- Ideally, coffee should be decaffeinated (see page 49). However, if you can't face a day without your morning jolt of java, then go for it, but make sure you limit it to one cup per day. Never add sugar—use sweeteners instead. Use only 1% or skim milk.

- Tea is acceptable, as it has considerably less caffeine than coffee.

LUNCH

Because lunch is the meal most of us eat outside the home, it can be the most problematic, limited by time, budget, and availability. But there appears to be a trend toward brown-bagging lunch, which gives you considerably more control over your food options. Here are some practical guidelines for when you bring lunch. If your preference is eating out at a restaurant or fast-food joint, turn to chapter 7, Eating Out.

PROTEIN

	● RED LIGHT	● YELLOW LIGHT	● GREEN LIGHT
meat*/ poultry*/ seafood*/ eggs/meat substitutes	Bacon (regular) Bologna Bratwurst Ground beef (regular—more than 20% fat) Hamburgers Hot dogs Pastrami (beef) Processed meats Salami Sausages	Chicken thighs, wings, and legs (skinless) Ground beef (lean— 10–20% fat) Lamb (lean cuts) Pork (lean cuts) Tofu (firm) Turkey bacon Whole eggs (preferably omega-3)	Beef (lean cuts) Chicken breast (skinless) Deli meats (lean) Egg Beaters Egg whites Ground beef (extra lean— 10% or less fat) Liquid eggs Pastrami (turkey) Pork tenderloin Seafood, fresh or frozen (no batter or breading), or canned (in water) Smoked salmon Tofu (soft) Turkey breast (skinless) Veal

*Limit serving size (see page 25).

PROTEIN (continued)

	RED LIGHT	YELLOW LIGHT	GREEN LIGHT
dairy	Cheese (regular) Cottage cheese (whole or 2%) Cream cheese (regular) Ice cream (regular) Milk (whole or 2%) Sour cream (regular) Yogurt (whole or 2%)	Cheese (low-fat) Cream cheese (light) Ice cream (low-fat) Milk (1%) Sour cream (light) Yogurt (low-fat with sugar)	Cheese (fat-free) Cottage cheese (1% or fat-free) Cream cheese (nonfat) Extra-low-fat cheese (e.g., Laughing Cow Light, Boursin Light) Flavored yogurt (fat-free with sweetener) Ice cream (low-fat and no added sugar)* Milk (skim) Sour cream (1% or fat-free) Soy milk (plain, low-fat)

CARBOHYDRATES

	RED LIGHT	YELLOW LIGHT	GREEN LIGHT
breads/ grains	Bagels Baguettes and other crusty white breads Biscuits Cake/cookies Croissants and pastries	Crispbreads (with fiber; e.g., Ryvita High Fiber) Pita (whole wheat) Tortillas (whole wheat)	Crispbreads (with high fiber; e.g., Wasa Fiber)* Homemade Apple Bran Muffins (see page 86)

*Limit serving size (see page 25).

	🔴 RED LIGHT	⚪ YELLOW LIGHT	🔵 GREEN LIGHT
breads/ grains (continued)	Croutons Doughnuts Gnocchi Hamburger/ hot dog buns Macaroni and cheese Muffins (commercial) Noodles (canned or instant) Pancakes/waffles Pasta filled with cheese and/or meat Pizza Rice (instant, short grain, white) Tortillas (regular) White sandwich bread	Whole-grain breads (less than 3g fiber/slice)	Pasta, any shape (use whole wheat or protein-enriched if available), cooked al dente* Pita (high fiber) Quinoa (and other whole grains) Rice (basmati, brown, long-grain, wild)* Whole-grain, high-fiber bread (at least 3g fiber per slice)*
fruits/ vegetables (fresh/ frozen/ dried/ canned)	Applesauce containing sugar Canned fruit in syrup (all) Cantaloupe Dried fruit (most)** Fava beans French fries Melons	Apricots (dried)** Apricots (fresh) Artichokes Bananas Beets Corn Fruit cocktail in juice Kiwi	Apples Applesauce (unsweetened) Arugula Asparagus Avocado (¼ of the fruit) Beans (green/wax) Bell peppers Blackberries Blueberries

*Limit serving size (see page 25).
**You may use a modest amount of dried fruit for baking.

CARBOHYDRATES (continued)

	● RED LIGHT	● YELLOW LIGHT	● GREEN LIGHT
fruits/ vegetables (fresh/ frozen/ dried/ canned) (continued)	Parsnips Potatoes (instant, mashed, or baked) Raisins** Rutabaga	Mangoes Papaya Pineapple Pomegranates Potatoes (boiled) Squash Sweet potatoes Yams	Broccoli Brussels sprouts Cabbage Carrots Cauliflower Celery Cherries Cucumbers Eggplant Grapefruit Grapes Leeks Lemons Lettuce Mushrooms Olives* Onions Oranges Peaches Pears Peas Peppers (hot) Pickles Plums Potatoes (boiled small, preferably new)* Radishes Raspberries Snow peas Spinach Strawberries Tomatoes Zucchini

*Limit serving size (see page 25).
**You may use a modest amount of dried fruit for baking.

FATS/CONDIMENTS/NUTS

● RED LIGHT	● YELLOW LIGHT	● GREEN LIGHT
Butter	Corn oil	Almonds*
Hard margarine	Mayonnaise (light)	Canola oil*
Ketchup		Cashews*
Mayonnaise (regular)	Natural peanut butter (100% peanuts)	Hazelnuts*
Peanut butter (regular and light)	Nuts, except those listed as green-light	Hummus
		Macadamia nuts*
Salad dressings (bottled, regular)	Salad dressings (bottled, light)	Mayonnaise (fat-free)
Tropical oils (such as palm and coconut)	Soft margarine (nonhydroge-nated)	Mustard
		Olive oil*
Vegetable shortening	Vegetable oils	Pistachios*
	Walnuts	Salad dressings (low-fat, low sugar)
		Soft margarine (nonhydroge-nated, light; e.g., Promise Light)*
		Vinaigrette

SOUPS

● RED LIGHT	● YELLOW LIGHT	● GREEN LIGHT
All cream-based soups	Canned chicken noodle	Canned chunky bean and vegetable soups (e.g., Campbell's Healthy Request)
Canned black bean	Canned lentil	
Canned green pea	Canned tomato	Homemade soups with green-light ingredients
Canned puréed vegetable		
Canned split pea		

*Limit serving size (see page 25).

THE BROWN-BAG OPTION

Bringing your lunch to work is the easiest way to ensure that you eat green-light. And there are other advantages to brown-bagging it, besides avoiding the temptation of a red-light lunch out: It's cheaper and it gives you extra downtime.

Sandwiches

Sandwiches are the lunchtime staple, and it's no wonder: They're portable and easy to make, and they offer endless variety. Sandwiches can also be a dietary disaster, but if you follow the suggestions below, you can keep yours green-light.

- Always use whole-grain, high-fiber bread (minimum of 3 grams of fiber per slice).

- Sandwiches should be served open-faced. Either pack components separately and assemble just before eating, or make your sandwich with a "lettuce lining" that helps keep the bread from getting soggy.

- Include at least three vegetables, such as lettuce, tomato, red or green bell pepper, cucumber, sprouts, or onion. Instead of spreading the bread with butter or margarine, use mustard or hummus.

- Add up to 4 ounces of cooked lean meat or fish or lean deli meats. If you make tuna or chicken salad, use fat-free or low-fat mayonnaise or low-fat salad dressing and celery. Mix canned salmon with malt vinegar or fresh lemon.

If your preference is to purchase your sandwiches, then select those that are made with whole-grain, high-fiber bread. Remove the top layer of bread and eat the sandwich open-faced. Watch out for mayonnaise—it's often a major component in egg, chicken, and tuna salads. Always ask for no mayo—unless it's fat-free or low-fat. Also request no butter or margarine on bread. Hummus and mustard are good alternatives.

A popular alternative to sandwiches are wraps. Ask for a whole-wheat pita or low-carb tortilla. While regular tortillas are red-light, low-carb tortillas with high fiber and low fat are acceptable. They're also great for brown bagging. If you choose pita bread, have it split in half so you get only a single layer.

Salads

Invest in a variety of reusable plastic containers so you can bring salads to work. Keep a supply of green-light vinaigrette on hand and wash greens ahead of time; store in paper towels in plastic bags. You'll find that salads are a creative way to use up leftovers with a minimum of fuss.

SNACKS

Keep your digestive system busy and your energy up with three snacks daily. They are an important part of the G.I. Diet. But I'm afraid you'll have to avoid the customary choices like muffins, cookies, and chips, all high-G.I. foods that are fat- and calorie-dense. Two hours after eating them, you've added a few more fat cells and are feeling hungry again. These foods are just not worth the consequences!

You might also want to explore the world of high-protein bars, but be careful when choosing, as most of them are full of cereal and sugar. The ones to look for have a high protein content—at least 12 to 15 grams per 50- to 60-gram bar. Half a Balance Bar or Zone Bar is an excellent snack. Check labels carefully, and remember the serving size is *half* a 50- to 60-gram bar.

If you bake your own low-G.I. muffins and granola bars, they also make good snacks. You can freeze a batch or two and reheat them in the microwave. See chapter 5, Meal Ideas, for delicious recipes.

Though many snacks and desserts are billed as fat- and sugar-free, they are in fact high-G.I. because often all they contain are

SNACKS

● RED LIGHT	● YELLOW LIGHT	● GREEN LIGHT
Bagels	Bananas	Extra-low-fat cheese (e.g., Laughing Cow Light, Boursin Light)
Candy	Dark chocolate (70% cocoa)*	
Cookies		
Crackers	Ice cream (low-fat)	Flavored yogurt (fat-free with sweetener)
Doughnuts	Nuts, except those listed as green-light	
French fries		Fresh fruit (most)
Granola bars (commercial)	Popcorn (microwave light)	Fresh vegetables (most)
Ice cream (regular)		Frozen yogurt (½ cup; low-fat)
Jell-O		
Milk chocolate		Hazelnuts*
Muffins (commercial)		High-protein bars**
Popcorn (microwave, pre-popped)		Homemade Apple Bran Muffins (see page 86)
Potato chips		
Pretzels		Homemade Granola Bars (see page 87)
Pudding		
Raisins		Ice cream (low-fat and no added sugar)*
Rice cakes		
Sorbet	Almonds*	
Tortilla chips	Applesauce (unsweetened)	Macadamia nuts*
Trail mix		
White bread	Canned peaches or pears in juice	Pickles
	Cashews*	Pistachios*
	Cheese (fat-free)	Pumpkin seeds
	Cottage cheese (1% or fat-free)	Sugar-free hard candies
		Sunflower seeds

*Limit serving size (see page 25).

**Warning: Most so-called nutrition bars are high-G.I. and high-calorie, with a lot of quick-fix carbs. Look for 50- to 60-gram bars, with 12 to 15 grams of protein per bar. (Balance bars are a good choice.)

highly processed grains: for example, fat- and sugar-free puddings and Jell-O and fat- and sugar-free muffins.

Try to incorporate a balance of carbohydrates, fats, and proteins into each snack. For example, have a few nuts; nonfat, sugar-free yogurt with a piece of fruit; or Laughing Cow Light Cheese with celery sticks. Though achieving this balance with each snack can be difficult, especially when you're away from home, the effort is worth it.

DINNER

Traditionally, dinner is the main meal of the day—and the one where most of us blow our diet to shreds. Unlike breakfast and lunch, dinner doesn't usually have any time or availability constraints (although juggling our schedules along with our families' can sometimes make this a moot point).

The typical American dinner comprises three things: meat or fish; potato, pasta, or rice; and vegetables. Together, these foods provide carbohydrates, proteins, and fats, along with other minerals and vitamins essential to our health. For tips on cooking the green-light way, see pages 60 to 63.

PROTEIN

	● RED LIGHT	● YELLOW LIGHT	● GREEN LIGHT
meat*/ poultry*/ seafood*/ eggs/meat substitutes	Bacon (regular) Bratwurst Ground beef (regular—more than 20% fat) Hamburgers Hot dogs	Chicken thighs, wings, and legs (skinless) Ground beef (lean—10–20% fat) Lamb (lean cuts) Pork (lean cuts)	Beef (lean cuts) Chicken breast (skinless) Deli meats (lean) Egg Beaters Egg whites

*Limit serving size (see page 25).

PROTEIN (continued)

	● RED LIGHT	○ YELLOW LIGHT	● GREEN LIGHT
meat*/ poultry*/ seafood*/ eggs/meat substitutes (continued)	Processed meats Sausages	Tofu (firm) Turkey bacon Whole eggs (preferably omega-3)	Ground beef (extra lean— 10% or less fat) Liquid eggs Pork tenderloin Seafood, fresh or frozen (no batter or breading), or canned (in water) Tofu (soft) Turkey breast (skinless) Veal
dairy	Cheese (regular) Cottage cheese (whole or 2%) Ice cream (regular) Milk (whole or 2%) Sour cream (regular) Yogurt (whole or 2%)	Cheese (low-fat) Ice cream (low-fat) Milk (1%) Sour cream (light) Yogurt (low-fat with sugar)	Cheese (fat-free) Cottage cheese (1% or fat-free) Extra-low-fat cheese (e.g., Laughing Cow Light, Boursin Light) Flavored yogurt (fat-free with sweetener) Frozen yogurt (½ cup; low-fat) Ice cream (low-fat and no added sugar)* Milk (skim) Sour cream (1% or fat-free) Soy milk (plain, low-fat)

*Limit serving size (see page 25).

CARBOHYDRATES

	● RED LIGHT	● YELLOW LIGHT	● GREEN LIGHT
breads/ grains	Bagels	Couscous (whole wheat)	Crispbreads (with high fiber; e.g., Wasa Fiber)*
	Baguettes and other crusty white breads	Crispbreads (with fiber; e.g., Ryvita High Fiber)	Homemade Apple Bran Muffins (see page 86)
	Biscuits	Pita (whole wheat)	
	Cake/cookies	Sourdough bread	Pasta, any shape (use whole wheat or protein-enriched if available), cooked al dente*
	Corn bread	Tortillas (whole wheat)	
	Couscous		
	Croissants and pastries	Whole-grain breads (less than 3g fiber/slice)	Quinoa and other whole grains
	Doughnuts		
	Gnocchi		Rice (basmati, brown, long-grain, wild)*
	Hamburger/ hot dog buns		
	Macaroni and cheese		Whole-grain, high-fiber bread (at least 3g fiber per slice)*
	Muffins (commercial)		
	Noodles (canned or instant)		
	Pancakes/ waffles		
	Pasta filled with cheese and/or meat		
	Pizza		
	Rice (instant, short-grain white)		
	Tortillas (regular)		
	White sandwich bread		

*Limit serving size (see page 25).

CARBOHYDRATES (continued)

	RED LIGHT	YELLOW LIGHT	GREEN LIGHT
fruits/ vegetables (fresh/ frozen/ dried)	Applesauce containing sugar	Apricots (dried)**	Arugula
	Dried fruit (most)**	Apricots (fresh)	Asparagus
	Fava beans	Bananas	Avocado (¼ of fruit)
	French fries	Beets	Beans (green/wax)
	Melons	Corn	Bell peppers
	Parsnips	Kiwi	Broccoli
	Potatoes (instant, mashed, or baked)	Mangoes	Brussels sprouts
	Raisins**	Papaya	Cabbage
	Rutabagas	Pineapple	Carrots
		Pomegranates	Cauliflower
		Potatoes (boiled)	Celery
		Squash	Cucumbers
		Sweet potatoes	Eggplant
		Yams	Leeks
			Lettuce
			Mushrooms
		Apples	Olives*
		Applesauce (unsweetened)	Onions
		Blackberries	Peas
		Blueberries	Peppers (hot)
		Cherries	Pickles
		Grapefruit	Potatoes (boiled small, preferably new)*
		Grapes	Radishes
		Lemons	Snow peas
		Oranges	Spinach
		Peaches	Tomatoes
		Pears	Zucchini
		Plums	
		Raspberries	
		Strawberries	

*Limit serving size (see page 25).

**You may use a modest amount of dried fruit for baking.

FATS/CONDIMENTS/NUTS

● RED LIGHT	○ YELLOW LIGHT	● GREEN LIGHT
Butter	Corn oil	Almonds*
Hard margarine	Mayonnaise (light)	Canola oil*
Lard	Natural peanut butter (100% peanuts)	Cashews*
Mayonnaise (regular)	Nuts, except those listed as green-light	Hazelnuts*
Peanut butter (regular and light)	Salad dressings (bottled, light)	Macadamia nuts*
Salad dressings (bottled, regular)	Soft margarine (nonhydrogenated)	Mayonnaise (fat-free)
Tropical oils (such as palm and coconut)	Vegetable oils	Olive oil*
Vegetable shortening	Walnuts	Pistachios*
		Salad dressings (low-fat, low-sugar)
		Soft margarine (nonhydrogenated, light; e.g., Promise Light)*
		Vinaigrette

SOUPS

● RED LIGHT	○ YELLOW LIGHT	● GREEN LIGHT
All cream-based soups	Canned chicken noodle	Canned chunky bean and vegetable (e.g., Campbell's Healthy Request)
Canned black bean	Canned lentil	Homemade soups with green-light ingredients
Canned green pea	Canned tomato	Miso
Canned puréed vegetable		
Canned split pea		

*Limit serving size (see page 25).

Meat/Seafood

- Most red meat contains saturated (bad) fat, so it's important to buy lean cuts and trim off *all* the visible fat. A loin steak trimmed to only ¼ inch of fat can have up to twice the fat of a steak that has been completely trimmed. Obviously, some cuts of meat have an intrinsically higher fat content, and these should be avoided. The best buys are top round beef, veal, and pork tenderloin. Check with your butcher if you're not sure which cuts have the lowest fat content.

- Chicken and turkey breasts are excellent choices *provided all the skin is removed.* Skinless thighs, wings, and legs are higher in fat and are therefore yellow-light.

- Seafood is also an excellent choice unless it's been breaded. Certain fish, such as salmon, have a relatively high oil content, but this oil is extremely beneficial to your health, especially your heart health.

- In terms of quantity, the best measure for meat or fish is your palm. The portion should be about the size of the palm of your hand and about as thick. Another good visual is a pack of cards— so my friends with small palms tell me!

Meat Substitutes

There are an increasing number of green-light alternatives to animal protein. Beans and tofu are excellent sources of protein, and you don't have to be a vegetarian to enjoy them. Beans are, in fact, nearly the perfect food, as they not only contain protein but also are low in fat and high in fiber. And they make a great addition to salads and soups.

Though tofu may not be very exciting by itself, it takes on the flavors of whatever seasonings and sauces it is cooked with. Choose soft tofu, which has up to a third less fat than the firm variety.

Potatoes

- The G.I. rating of potatoes ranges from moderate to high, depending on the type and how they're cooked and served. In the lowest G.I. category are boiled small, preferably new potatoes, two to three per serving. All other versions are strictly red light.

Pasta

- Serving size is critical. Pasta should be a side dish and not form the base of the meal. In other words, it should take up only a quarter of your plate. Whole wheat pasta, available in your local supermarket, is preferable. Allow ¾ cup cooked pasta per serving.

Rice

- Rice has a broad G.I. range. The best choices are basmati, wild, brown, or long-grain. These rices contain a starch, amylose, that breaks down more slowly than the starch in other rices. Again, serving size is critical. Allow 3 tablespoons of dry rice per serving, or ⅔ cup cooked.

Vegetables/Salad

- This is where you can go wild. Eat as many vegetables and as much salad as you like. In fact, this should be the backbone of your meal. Virtually all vegetables are ideal. Try to have a side salad with your daily dinner.

- Watch out for salad dressings. Use only low-fat, low-sugar ones, or a small amount of olive oil with vinegar or lemon juice. Check the sugar content of bottled dressings, as manufacturers often bump up the sugar as they reduce the fat.

- Serve two or three varieties of vegetables for dinner. Family-size frozen bags of mixed, unseasoned vegetables are as nutritious as fresh, and they're inexpensive and convenient.

Soups

• A chunky bean or vegetable soup followed by fish or chicken makes an ideal dinner. But beware of cream-based or puréed vegetable soups. They are high in fat and heavily processed, and therefore red-light all the way.

Note: Because of their high-temperature processing, commercial soups have a higher G.I. rating than those that are cooked from scratch.

Desserts

This is one of the most troublesome issues in any weight-control program. Desserts usually look and taste great, but they tend to be loaded with sugar and fat—a real guilt-inducing situation! As the last course in most meals, desserts often fall into the "should I or shouldn't I?" category.

The good news is that dessert should be a part of your meal. There is a broad range of green-light alternatives that taste great and are good for you. Virtually any fruit qualifies (though hold off on the bananas and raisins), and there are numerous low-fat, low-sugar dairy products such as yogurt and ice cream. You won't be eating apple pie à la mode, but you could be enjoying unsweetened applesauce with yogurt, or even a meringue with fresh or frozen berries.

BEVERAGES

Since 70 percent of our body is made up of water, it's hardly surprising that drinking water is an important part of any dietary program. Most dieticians recommend that we drink eight glasses of fluid per day.

If you drink eight glasses of water, you'll end up consuming a great deal more than that, because we take in fluids without even being conscious of it. Add all the other liquids you consume, such as diet soft drinks and the milk you put on your cereal, along with the water that makes up a great deal of the bulk of most fruits and vegetables, and you'll easily take in several cups a day without even trying. So the rule of thumb is this: Drink at least a glass of water before each of your three main meals and with each snack. Because liquids don't trip satiety mechanisms, it's simply a waste to take in calories through them. So what to drink?

Water

The cheapest and best beverage choice is plain water. Try to drink an 8-ounce glass of water *before* each meal for a couple of reasons. First, having your stomach partly filled with liquid before the meal means that you'll feel full more quickly, thus reducing the temptation to overeat. Second, you won't be tempted to "wash down" your food before it's been sufficiently chewed, thus upsetting your digestive system.

Soft Drinks

If water is too boring for you, go for sugar-free soft drinks, preferably also caffeine-free (see "Coffee," below), in moderation. Remember, the sugar in a drink is less satisfying than an equal quantity of sugar in food, so don't waste your calorie-intake quota.

Skim Milk

My personal beverage preference is skim milk, at least with breakfast and lunch. It's an ideal green-light food, and since most lunches tend to be protein deficient, drinking skim milk is a good way to make up some of the shortfall.

Coffee

The principal problem with coffee is caffeine. Caffeine effectively encourages appetite. If you can't start your day without a cup, by all means go ahead, but limit yourself to one cup a day. An alternative is decaffeinated coffee—no hardship, given the delicious range of decaffeinated options available today.

As an experiment, I asked a group of dinner guests whether they preferred caffeinated or decaffeinated coffee. It split about fifty-fifty. I then served top-quality decaffeinated coffee to everyone and asked how they liked it. I received more applause from those who had asked for caffeinated than from the dedicated decaf aficionados! I rest my case.

Tea

Tea has considerably less caffeine than coffee. Both black and green teas also contain an antioxidant property that appears to carry a significant heart health benefit. In fact, there are higher quantities of flavonoids (antioxidants) in tea than in any vegetable tested. Two cups of black or green tea have the same amount of antioxidants as seven cups of orange juice or twenty of apple juice. Maybe my 99-year-old mother and her tea-drinking cronies are on to something!

So tea in moderation is fine. If you are looking for alternative teas that are completely caffeine-free, there is a wide variety of decaf, flavored herbal, and fruit options, though they don't have the antioxidant characteristics of black and green teas.

Iced tea is good, too, as long as no sugar is added. But pre-sweetened teas, whether bottled or homemade, are red-light.

Fruit Drinks/Juices

Fruit drinks contain large amounts of sugar, are calorie-dense, and definitely belong on the red-light list.

Fruit juices, which are 100 percent pure juice, are preferable, but as we discussed earlier, it is always better to eat the fruit or vegetable rather than drink its juice. Juice contains less nutrition and more calories than the original fruit or vegetable and has a higher G.I. Remember, the more work your body has to do to break down food, the better.

Alcohol

I'm sure this is the section that many readers fast-forward to. Well, it's a good news/bad news story. The good news is that alcohol in moderation—particularly red wine—is not only acceptable, but can even be good for your health. Red wine is a particularly rich source of antioxidants, especially flavonoids. We'll discuss moderation in chapter 6, Phase II.

The bad news is that alcohol in general is a disaster for weight control. Alcohol is easily metabolized by the body, which means increased insulin production, a drop in blood sugar levels, and demand from the body for more alcohol or food to boost those sagging sugar levels. This is a vicious cycle that can wreak havoc on your weight-loss plans. To make things worse, most alcoholic drinks are loaded with empty calories.

So NO ALCOHOL AT ALL in Phase I.

THE FAMILY

One of the most frequent questions I'm asked is whether the G.I. Diet is suitable for all members of the family, including children—and indeed it is. Phase II is a healthy way to eat for everyone, even if they don't need to lose any weight. Phase I is recommended for anyone who needs to reduce, but if you think your child may be overweight, *it is critical that you get your doctor's confirmation*. Kids often put on weight prior to a growth spurt, and it's not something you should necessarily worry about. However, childhood obesity in this country has tripled over the past twenty-five years, so it's important to introduce children to good eating habits. Children should always eat a nutritious breakfast (not sugary cereals), lunch, dinner, and snacks made up of green- and yellow-light foods. Fresh fruit, vegetables, chicken, fish, yogurt, whole-grain high-fiber bread, pasta, oatmeal, and nuts are all kid-friendly foods that will see to their nutritional needs. Remember that growing children need sufficient fat in their diet—the good kind found in nuts, fish, and vegetable oils.

If your doctor agrees that your child is overweight, introduce him or her to the Phase I way of eating. Don't put pressure on children to lose weight—simply *encourage* healthy food choices. And allow them to enjoy special treats on holidays and occasions such as birthdays and Halloween.

VEGETARIANS

I was surprised at the number of vegetarians who wrote to me asking whether the G.I. Diet was right for them. Most vegetarians I know don't need to lose weight. But if you don't eat meat and you need to drop some pounds, the G.I. Diet can certainly be the program for you. Just continue to substitute vegetable protein for animal protein—something you've been doing all along. However, because most vegetable protein sources, such as beans, are encased in fiber, your digestive system may not be getting the maximum protein benefit. So try to add easily digestible protein boosters like tofu and soy protein powder.

You will find several vegetarian recipes in chapter 5, Meal Ideas, as well as suggestions on how to convert some recipes with meat to meatless.

---

to sum up

1. In Phase I, eat exclusively green-light foods, i.e., those with a low glycemic, saturated fat, and calorie rating.

2. Eat three principal meals of equal nutritional value per day, plus three snacks.

3. Drink lots of water, including an 8-ounce glass before each meal and snack. Avoid caffeine or alcohol until Phase II!

4. Moderation and common sense are your guides for determining serving portions.

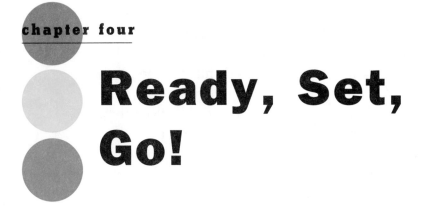

chapter four

Ready, Set, Go!

READY

By now, I hope you understand the principles of the G.I. Diet and are totally convinced that the plan is going to work for you for the rest of your life. All that's left is to take the plunge. This is what I call the READY stage, and it is perhaps the most difficult part of the journey.

Important note: If you have any medical condition or are pregnant, check with your doctor before starting this or any other diet plan.

The best advice I can give comes from my own experience. I knew I had to lose 20 pounds to take me to my 22 BMI target weight. On the advice of a friend, I gathered together a number of books (diet books!) and piled them on my bathroom scale until they totaled 20 pounds. I then put them in a backpack and carried them around the house one Sunday morning. By noon, the weight was really bugging me. What a relief it was to take the bag off my back! So the question was, did I want to carry that excess 20 pounds of fat around with me each and every day, or lose it and gain the sense of lightness and freedom I experienced after the backpack came off?

I urge you to try the same exercise. Identify how much weight you want to lose by using the BMI chart on pages 16 to 17. Rather than bundling up books, which can be rather bulky (especially if you have a lot of weight to lose), fill some empty plastic bottles or jugs with water to equal that weight, and carry them around in shopping bags for a few hours. Remember, that's the excess weight you are permanently carrying around with you. No wonder you feel exhausted! That's one of the principal benefits of the G.I. Diet: Not only will you look and feel great, but you will rediscover all that energy and zip you had in your teens and twenties, which you thought had been lost forever.

SET

Wondering what to do first? Well, let me suggest that you proceed in the following manner:

1. Baseline

Before you do anything else, get your vital statistics on record. Measuring progress is a great motivator. On page 155 you'll find a detachable log sheet to keep in the bathroom so you can record your weekly progress. Two measurements are key. The first is weight. Always weigh yourself at the same time of day, because a meal or bowel movement can throw off your weight by a couple of pounds. First thing in the morning, before you eat breakfast, is a good time. The other important measurement is your waist. Measure at your natural waistline—usually just above the navel— while standing in a relaxed, normal posture. The tape should be snug but not indenting the skin.

Record both measurements on the bathroom log. I've added a "Comments" column to the log sheet, where you can note how you're feeling or any unusual events in the past week that might have some bearing on your progress.

2. Pantry

Clear all red- and yellow-light products out of your pantry, fridge, and freezer. Don't compromise; give them to a food bank or to your neighbors. If these items are not around, you won't be tempted to eat or drink them.

3. Shopping

Stock up on products that get a green light. You'll find a detachable shopping list on page 150 to take with you to the grocery store. After a couple of trips, selecting the right products will become second nature.

Although I've tried to provide a broad range of products, I could not hope to cover all the thousands of brands available in most supermarkets. As a result, I've listed foods by their generic name; for instance, "oatmeal," not "Quaker Oats." In today's competitive marketplace, most brands in any given category have similar formulations, so you will usually choose based on quality and taste. In the rare instances where there may be some variations in content between brands—bread is a good example—you may want to check out the nutrition labels. Look for six key numbers:

1. **Serving size:** Is this realistic? Often manufacturers who are concerned about the fat, cholesterol, or calorie content of that product will identify a serving size that's smaller than is realistic. You'll see this on the labels of many high-sugar cereals.

2. **Calories:** Remember that this number is based on the serving size, which should be realistic. The lower, the better.

3. **Fat:** Look for the brand with less fat per serving, particularly trans- and saturated fat.

4. **Fiber:** Since fibrous foods have a lower G.I., look for products with the highest number of fiber grams per serving.

5. Sugar: Choose brands that are lower in sugar. Watch out for products advertised as low-fat wherein the manufacturer has bumped up the sugar content to make up for any perceived loss of taste. Yogurts and cereals are good examples. Sugars are sometimes listed as dextrose, glucose, fructose, or sucrose; regardless of the form, it's sugar. Similarly, sugar alcohols—easily identifiable because they end in "-tol" (such as sorbitol or maltitol)—contain around 60 to 70 percent of the calories that sugar contains. But as they are correspondingly less sweet, manufacturers tend to boost their levels; thus there's no net calorie savings over sugar. So avoid them.

6. Sodium (salt): Sodium increases water retention, which doesn't help when you're trying to lose weight. It also contributes to premenstrual bloating in women and is a factor in hypertension (high blood pressure). Combine high blood pressure with excess weight and you substantially raise your risk of heart disease and stroke. We currently consume more than twice the amount of salt recommended for a healthy diet.

Basically, when you choose between brands, choose the ones that offer lower calories, fat (especially saturated), sugar, and sodium and that are higher in fiber. This is the formula for all green-light products: They have a low G.I., are low in saturated fat, and are calorie-light. By eating these foods, you will reduce your caloric intake without going hungry.

You will be buying considerably more fruit and vegetables than previously, so be a little daring and try some varieties that are new to you. There's a wonderful world of fresh and frozen produce just waiting for you to enjoy! Remember, frozen produce has the same nutritional value as fresh.

Caution: Don't go food shopping on an empty stomach, or you'll end up buying items that don't belong on the G.I. Diet!

GO!

Now that the difficult part is done, it's smooth sailing from here. Don't be surprised if you lose more than one pound per week during the first few weeks as your body adjusts to the new regimen. Some of that weight will be water, not fat (remember that 70 percent of our body weight is water).

Don't worry if from time to time you "fall off the wagon," eating or drinking with friends and going outside the program. That's the real world, and though it will marginally delay your target date, it's more important that you not feel overly constrained. You should aim to live about 90 percent within the program and 10 percent outside. When on the program, you'll feel better and more energized, and rarely deprived. However, try to keep these lapses to a minimum in Phase I; you'll be able to allow yourself more leeway once you have achieved your target weight.

If you want further proof or reassurance that your new way of eating is really working, try this test. After a couple of months on the G.I. Diet, break all the rules and have a lunch consisting of a whole pizza with the works, a bread roll, and a beer or regular soft drink. While you're at it, finish up with a slice of pie. I'll spare you the ice cream.

I did just that, and by about three in the afternoon, I could hardly stay awake. I felt listless and worn out. I hadn't planned on eating so much but got caught up in a fellow employee's farewell lunch. The reason for my afternoon fatigue (which you've likely figured out for yourself) was the combination of high-G.I. foods (pizza, bread roll, beer, and pie), which led to a rapid spike in my blood sugar level. The resulting rush of insulin drained this sugar from my blood and caused my sugar levels to drop precipitously, leaving my brain and muscles starved of energy—in a hypoglycemic state. No wonder I couldn't keep my eyes open.

Though we will be talking more extensively about motivation in chapter 9, here are some tips to keep you motivated, especially when your resolve starts flagging (as it inevitably will from time to time):

1. Maintain a weekly progress log (see page 155 for a removable log sheet). Nothing is more motivating than success.

2. Set up a reward system. Buy yourself a small gift when you achieve a predetermined weight-loss goal—perhaps a gift for every three pounds lost.

3. Identify family members or friends who will be your cheerleaders. Make them active participants in your plan. Even better, find a friend who will join the plan for mutual support.

4. Avoid acquaintances and haunts that may encourage your old behaviors. You know who and where I mean!

5. Try adding what a friend calls a special "spa day" to your week—a day when you are especially good with your program. This gives you some extra credit in your weight-loss account to draw on when the inevitable relapse occurs.

6. Sign up for the free G.I. Diet newsletter to learn from readers' experiences and keep up-to-date on the latest developments in diet and health. Details are at www.gidiet.com.

To give you some encouragement and motivation as you start your journey, I'll leave you with the words of a few other readers who've found success with the G.I. Diet:

> *"I have PCOS [polycystic ovary syndrome] and insulin resistance. Weight has ALWAYS been an issue for me. I was bulimic a good part of my high school years. I got married and that year, with my husband's support, overcame the bulimia but gained about 80 pounds. Over the following six years we tried so desperately to get pregnant, and it just didn't happen. Lo and*

behold, this diet managed to do what fertility drugs, thyroid pills, and herbal supplements could not, and after the hardest six years of my life, I now have the most beautiful baby boy ever born. Thank you so much!" —Kristina

"This is, without a doubt, the most expensive diet I have ever been on. After a short three months, I've lost 30 pounds. I'm approaching 200 pounds for the first time in years, and I have to completely replace my wardrobe! My suits don't fit anymore and all my pants are beyond 'too big.' The best part is I will have to replace everything again by December." —Brian

"I started this diet—I prefer to say new eating lifestyle— weighing in at 204 pounds and a size 22. In the year I have been following this plan I have gotten my weight down to 142 pounds and a size 10–12. I love this new me and I have gotten a lot of compliments. People always ask what my secret is and I go on and on about the book and the eating plan. I tell them that with this plan a lot of my cravings for high-carbohydrate foods have nearly vanished. I love this diet!" —Laurie

to sum up

1. Try the water bottle exercise (see page 54).
2. Record your baseline weight and waist measurement.
3. Clear the pantry, fridge, and freezer of all red- and yellow-light products. Replace with green-light products.
4. Follow the six motivational tips (facing page) and keep a record of your progress.
5. *Go for it!*

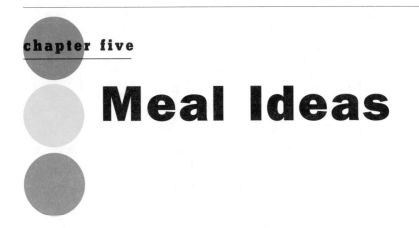

chapter five

Meal Ideas

Before looking at meal ideas, it is important that you get set up in the kitchen to cook the green-light way.

EQUIPMENT

The right equipment will help you retain the maximum nutritional benefit of your foods, as well as save you time. Every G.I. Diet kitchen should have the following:

Microwave Oven

Cooking food is really the first step in the digestive process—the longer food is cooked, the more "digestible" it becomes. As a result, cooking raises the G.I. of foods, as it does what your digestive system would otherwise be doing. Remember, it's important to have your body process food. Though I don't recommend always eating uncooked foods—ever tried eating a raw potato? It would take you a week to digest it!—I do suggest keeping cooking times to a minimum, or cooking only until food is done.

One of the best ways of doing this is with a microwave oven. Fresh or frozen vegetables can be cooked in minutes, helping to keep the G.I. low. It also preserves nutrients better than other methods because cooking time is minimal and little or no water is used (since microwaves vary, all cooking times I've given are approximate). Also good for thawing meats and warming leftovers, the microwave is your best green-light kitchen friend.

Nonstick Frying Pans

You should have two sizes, plus lids. They require little or no oil, and cleaning up is a cinch. We are big on stir-fries in our household, so these nonstick skillets get a lot of use.

Barbecue/Indoor Grill

Cooking meat and fish on either an outdoor or indoor grill is a good idea, as it allows any extra fat to drain away and always seems to make food taste better, too.

CONVERTING RECIPES

I have included green-light recipes for meals and snacks in this chapter. You don't necessarily have to use the recipes listed in this book, though. It's easy to make many of your own recipes green-light by following the guidelines below.

Green-Light Ingredients

First, ensure that all the ingredients in the recipe are green-light. If there are any red- or yellow-light ingredients, either omit or replace them with the green-light alternative. Some red- and yellow-light food can be used if the recipe calls for a very limited quantity, such as half a cup of wine in a dish that will serve six people, or a quarter cup of raisins in a salad for four. Full-flavored cheeses can also be used sparingly. For example, a tablespoon or two of grated Parmesan cheese sprinkled over a casserole will add flavor without too many calories. As long as the red- and yellow-light ingredients are used in very limited quantities and not as the core ingredients, they will not have a significant impact on the overall G.I. or green-light rating of the recipe.

Fiber

The fiber content of the recipe is critical. Fiber, both soluble and insoluble, is key to the overall G.I. rating of the recipe. The more, the better. If your recipe is light on fiber, consider adding fiber boosters such as oats, bran, whole grain, or beans.

Fat

Recipes should be low in fat, with little or no saturated fat. If a fat is called for, use vegetable oil. Canola and olive oil are your best choices, but use as little as possible, as all fats are calorie-dense. Cutting fat doesn't mean you have to cut flavor. Cream products can be replaced by fat-free yogurt, yogurt cheese (see the box on page 84), or fat-free sour cream. Use fat-free mayonnaise in tuna or chicken salad.

Try some new spices and flavored vinegars. Tomato salsa will spice up many foods without adding calories or fat, and fresh ginger adds life to stir-fries.

Sugar

Never add sugar or sugar-based ingredients such as corn syrup or molasses. There are some excellent sugar substitutes on the market. Our family's favorite is Splenda, which was developed from a sugar base but does not contain calories. It works well in cooking and baking. Measure it by volume (not weight) to effectively replace sugar. For example, 1 tablespoon of sugar equals 1 tablespoon of Splenda. Note that Splenda Brown Sugar Blend is 50 percent sugar and is therefore not recommended. Sugar Twin Granulated Brown is an acceptable alternative.

Protein

Be sure that the recipe contains sufficient protein, or that you are serving it alongside some protein to round out the meal. Protein helps slow the digestive process, which effectively lowers the G.I. of a recipe. It is also the one component that is often overlooked at mealtime, particularly in recipes for salads and snacks. Useful protein boosters are low-fat dairy products; whey powder; lean meats, poultry, and seafood; egg whites; and beans and soy-based foods, such as tofu and soy powders.

The following recipes are for the three principle meals and snacks. For many more green-light recipes, see *Living the G.I. Diet.*

BREAKFAST

The first meal of the day is an important one, and oatmeal is the king of breakfast food. It is low-G.I. and low-calorie, is easy to prepare in the microwave, and stays with you all morning. Always use large-flake, rolled, or steel-cut oats—not one-minute or instant oats, as they have already been considerably processed. The body has to work harder to metabolize rolled oats, and this slows the digestive process and leaves you feeling fuller longer.

Oatmeal can be endlessly varied by changing the flavor of the yogurt you add or by mixing in sliced fruit or berries. My wife's favorite way to eat oatmeal is with skim milk, unsweetened applesauce, sliced almonds, and sweetener. Following is a recipe for my favorite oatmeal. Top it off with an orange and a glass of skim milk, and you have a delicious breakfast that will stay with you all morning.

Oatmeal

1 serving

> *½ cup large-flake, rolled, or steel-cut oats*
> *1 cup water or skim milk*
> *½ to ¾ cup fat-free flavored yogurt with sweetener*
> *2 tablespoons sliced plain almonds*
> *Sliced fresh fruit or berries*

Place the oats in a microwave-safe bowl and cover with water or skim milk. Microwave the oats on medium power for 3 minutes. Mix in the yogurt, almonds, and some fresh fruit.

Homemade Muesli

2 servings

> *1 cup large-flake, rolled, or steel-cut oats*
> *¾ cup skim milk*
> *¾ cup fat-free flavored yogurt with sweetener*
> *2 tablespoons sliced plain almonds*
> *¾ cup berries or diced apple or pear*
> *Sweetener*

Place the oats in a bowl, cover them with the milk, and let soak in the refrigerator overnight. Add the yogurt, almonds, fruit, and sweetener to taste, and mix well.

Cold Cereal

1 serving

> ½ cup green-light cereal, such as All-Bran or Bran Buds
> ½ cup skim milk
> 2 tablespoons sliced plain almonds
> ¾ cup sliced peach or pear, or berries
> Sweetener

Place the cereal in a bowl and pour the milk over it. Top with the almonds and fruit and add sweetener to taste.

Variation: A tasty alternative is to add ½ cup flavored fat- and sugar-free yogurt and to cut back a little on the milk. Though these cereals are not a lot of fun in themselves, they are tasty when you add some fruit, nuts, and yogurt.

---

cooking with sweetener

Splenda, Sweet'N Low, and Equal (or their generic equivalents) can all be substituted for sugar. These sweeteners are available in several forms—individual packets, baking granules, liquid, and tablets. While packets are generally equivalent in sweetness to 2 teaspoons of sugar, the intensity of sweetness can vary depending on the brand and the form, so check the label. If you are sweetening a beverage or ready-to-eat meal, simply use your own taste as a guide. If you are substituting for sugar in baking, follow the instructions on the box or the product website.

On-the-Run Breakfast

1 serving

> *1 cup fresh fruit, such as blueberries or sliced apples, pears,*
> *   peaches, or strawberries*
> *½ cup cottage cheese (1% or fat-free)*
> *½ cup wheat bran, such as All-Bran or Bran Buds*
> *2 tablespoons sliced plain almonds*
> *1 slice toast, spread with 2 teaspoons soft margarine*
> *   (nonhydrogenated, light) and 1 tablespoon double-fruit,*
> *   low-sugar preserves*

Place the fruit in a bowl and top with the cottage cheese, wheat bran, and almonds. Serve the toast alongside, and enjoy with a cup of decaffeinated coffee or tea.

Basic Omelet and Variations

1 serving

Omelets are easy to make, and you can vary them by adding any number of fresh vegetables, a little cheese, and/or some meat. You'll find the ingredients for a basic omelet here, along with suggestions for making Italian, Mexican, vegetarian, and Western versions. Don't stop with these—using the proportions as a guide, you can add whatever green-light ingredients strike your fancy. To round out the meal, include a cup of fresh fruit and a glass of skim milk or ½ to ¾ cup of fat- and sugar-free yogurt.

> *Vegetable oil cooking spray (preferably canola or olive oil)*
> *½ cup liquid eggs or egg whites*
> *¼ cup skim milk*

Italian Omelet

½ cup sliced mushrooms
1 ounce grated skim mozzarella cheese
½ cup tomato purée
Chopped fresh or dried herbs, such as oregano or basil

Mexican Omelet

1 cup chopped red and green bell pepper
½ cup sliced mushrooms
½ cup canned beans, drained and rinsed
Hot sauce or chili powder, for sprinkling over the omelet
   (optional)

Vegetarian Omelet

1 cup small broccoli florets
½ cup sliced mushrooms
½ cup chopped red and green bell pepper
1 ounce grated skim-milk cheese

Western Omelet

1 cup chopped red and green bell pepper
1 small onion, chopped
2 slices Canadian bacon, lean deli ham,
   or skinless turkey breast, chopped
Red pepper flakes or cayenne pepper (optional),
   for sprinkling over the omelet

Omelet Preparation

1. Spray oil in a small nonstick skillet, then place it over medium heat.

2. If you're making an omelet with vegetables, add the mushrooms, bell pepper, broccoli, and/or onion and sauté until tender, about 5 minutes. Transfer the sautéed vegetables to a plate and cover with aluminum foil to keep warm.

3. Beat the eggs with the milk and pour them into the skillet. Cook over medium heat until the eggs start to firm up. Then, carefully flip the omelet. Spread the vegetables, cheese, beans, meat, tomato purée, and herbs of your choice over the omelet. Continue cooking until it is done to your liking.

4. If desired, sprinkle the omelet with hot sauce, chili powder, red pepper flakes, or cayenne, then serve.

Variation: Make scrambled eggs by stirring the eggs as they cook, adding any additional ingredients while the eggs are still soft.

LUNCH

If you are eating lunch out, refer to chapter 7, Eating Out, for helpful tips about restaurants, takeout, and fast-food options. However, brown bagging is an increasingly popular option. It allows you to control the ingredients and amount of fat used, and you save money at the same time. The following green-light lunch recipes can be bagged and brought to work. Just add fresh or canned fruit (in juice, not syrup) for dessert, and have a glass of water or skim milk. You'll feel full and energized for the afternoon.

Basic Salad

1 serving

*1 ½ cups torn or coarsely chopped lettuce and/or greens,
   such as romaine, leaf, Boston, or iceberg lettuce, mesclun,
   arugula, or watercress*
1 small carrot, grated
½ red, yellow, or green bell pepper, chopped
1 plum tomato, cut into wedges
½ cup sliced cucumber
¼ cup sliced red onion (optional)
Basic Vinaigrette (recipe follows)

Place the lettuce and/or greens, carrot, bell pepper, tomato, cucumber, and onion, if using, in a bowl and toss to mix. Pour about 1 tablespoon of the vinaigrette over the salad and toss to mix.

Variations: Salads are green-light with plenty of fiber, but they don't usually have a lot of protein. Adding 4 ounces of canned tuna, cooked salmon, tofu, beans, chickpeas, cooked chicken, or another lean meat will provide a delicious solution to the problem.

Pay attention to the salad dressing. If you want to use a store-bought dressing, look for low-fat with low sugar.

Basic Vinaigrette

4 servings

> 2 tablespoons vinegar, such as white or red wine, balsamic,
>   rice, or cider, or lemon juice
> 1 tablespoon extra-virgin olive oil or canola oil
> ½ teaspoon Dijon mustard
> Pinch of salt
> Pinch of black pepper
> Pinch of dried herbs, such as thyme, oregano, basil,
>   marjoram, or mint, or Italian seasoning

Place the vinegar, oil, mustard, salt, pepper, and herbs in a small bowl and whisk to combine.

Variation: Minced fresh herbs, such as Italian (flat) parsley or basil, make great additions to salads and vinaigrettes.

Storage: Both the salad and the vinaigrette can be prepared ahead and stored separately, covered, in the refrigerator for up to 2 days.

Salade Niçoise

1 serving

>2 *small new potatoes, boiled and quartered*
>1 *cup green beans, briefly cooked*
>1 *cup torn or coarsely chopped lettuce*
>1 *tablespoon Basic Vinaigrette (see facing page) or*
>   *store-bought low-fat mustard vinaigrette*
>2 *ounces tuna (canned in water), drained and flaked*
>1 *omega-3 egg, hard-boiled, peeled, and quartered*
>5 *pitted black olives*
>1 *medium tomato, quartered*
>1 *anchovy fillet (optional)*
>*Chopped fresh parsley*
>*Salt and black pepper*

Place the potatoes, beans, and lettuce in a bowl. Add the low-fat mustard vinaigrette and toss gently. Top with the tuna, egg, olives, tomato, and anchovy, if using. Sprinkle parsley on top, then season lightly with salt and pepper to taste.

Variation: Substitute grilled fresh fish for the canned tuna.

Waldorf Chicken and Rice Salad

1 serving

> ⅔ cup cooked basmati or brown rice
> 1 medium apple, chopped
> 1 or 2 stalks celery, chopped
> ¼ cup walnuts
> 4 ounces cooked chicken (page 75), chopped
> 1 tablespoon store-bought light buttermilk dressing

Place the rice, apple, celery, walnuts, and chicken in a bowl. Pour the buttermilk dressing on top and stir to mix. Keep refrigerated until lunch and enjoy.

Basic Pasta Salad Lunch

1 serving

> ½ to ¾ cup cooked whole wheat pasta
>   (spirals, shells, or similar shape)
> 1 cup chopped cooked vegetables
>   (such as broccoli, asparagus, bell peppers, or scallions)
> ¼ cup light tomato sauce or other low-fat or nonfat pasta sauce
> 4 ounces chopped cooked chicken (page 75) or other lean meat,
>   such as ground lean turkey

Place the pasta, vegetables, tomato sauce, and chicken in a bowl and stir to mix well. Refrigerate the salad, covered, until ready to use, then heat it in the microwave or serve chilled.

Variation: You can use the proportions here as a guide and vary the vegetables, sauce, and source of protein to suit your tastes and add variety to your pasta salad lunches.

sandwiches

The variations are endless, but here are some guidelines to make even the humble sandwich a convenient and filling green-light meal.

1. Always use 100 percent whole-grain, high-fiber bread with a minimum of 3 grams of fiber per slice.

2. During Phase I, sandwiches should be served open-faced.

3. Include at least three vegetables, such as lettuce, tomato, red or green bell pepper, cucumber, sprouts, or onion.

4. Use mustard or hummus as a spread on the bread. No regular mayonnaise or butter.

5. Add 4 ounces of cooked lean meat or fish.

6. Mix tuna or chopped cooked chicken with low-fat or fat-free mayonnaise or low-fat salad dressing and celery.

7. Mix canned salmon with malt vinegar (don't worry about bones)—a popular sandwich choice in Canada and the United Kingdom.

8. To help sandwiches stay fresh, not soggy, pack the components separately and assemble them just before eating, if possible.

Cottage Cheese and Fruit

1 serving

Perfect for a lunch on the run.

> *1 cup low-fat or fat-free cottage cheese*
> *1 cup chopped fresh fruit or fruit canned in juice,*
>   *such as peaches, apricots, or pears*

Place the cottage cheese and fruit in a plastic bowl with a fitted lid. Store in the refrigerator until lunchtime, then stir to mix. Enjoy.

Variation: Use a tablespoon of no-added-sugar fruit spread or preserves instead of the chopped fruit.

DINNER

All of the following ideas for meals are based on the G.I. Diet portion ratios discussed in chapter 3, Phase I. Vegetables should take up 50 percent of your plate and should always include at least one green vegetable, a mixture of at least two other vegetables, and a green salad. Meat, poultry, or fish should fill 25 percent of your plate, and rice, pasta, or potatoes should cover the remaining 25 percent.

I have based these meal ideas on typical family dinners, modifying them according to G.I. principles.

Poultry: Basic Preparation

1 serving

Naturally low in fat, cooked chicken or turkey breast can be used in dozens of ways, combined with a variety of herbs, spices, and vegetables to enhance its flavor. You'll find instructions for a basic green-light method of cooking poultry here, followed by three recipes that use the cooked meat. The proportions here are for one serving and can be multiplied as necessary for the recipes.

Vegetable oil cooking spray (preferably canola or olive oil)
4 ounces skinless, boneless chicken breast or turkey breast, whole, sliced, or cubed

1. Spray oil in a small nonstick skillet, then place it over medium-high heat.

2. Add the chicken or turkey breast and sauté until firm to the touch and no longer pink, about 4 minutes per side for 1 chicken breast or piece of turkey or 5 to 6 minutes for slices or cubes.

Asian Stir-Fry

2 servings

> *Vegetable oil cooking spray (preferably canola or olive oil)*
> *3 cups chopped mixed vegetables, such as carrots, cauliflower,*
>   *broccoli, mushrooms, and snow peas (see Note)*
> *1 teaspoon grated fresh ginger*
> *1 teaspoon soy sauce*
> *Black pepper*
> *8 ounces cooked skinless, boneless chicken breast or turkey breast*
>   *(page 75)*

1. Spray oil in a nonstick skillet, then place it over medium heat.

2. Add the mixed vegetables to the skillet and sauté until tender, about 5 minutes.

3. Add the ginger and soy sauce and stir to mix. Season to taste with pepper.

4. Add the cooked chicken or turkey and stir to mix. Let simmer until the chicken or turkey is heated through, about 2 minutes, then serve.

Variation: To put the stir-fry together even more quickly, use 2 to 3 teaspoons of a light, store-bought stir-fry sauce in place of the fresh ginger, soy sauce, and pepper.

Note: For color, add chopped mixed green, yellow, and red bell peppers. For convenience, use frozen mixed vegetables or frozen cut peppers.

Italian Chicken

2 servings

> *8 ounces sliced mushrooms*
> *1 medium onion, sliced*
> *1 can (18 ounces) chopped Italian tomatoes*
> *1 clove garlic, minced*
> *Chopped fresh or dried oregano and basil*
> *8 ounces cooked skinless, boneless chicken breast or turkey breast*
> *(page 75)*

1. Place the mushrooms, onion, and tomatoes in a saucepan. Stir in a little water, to prevent the tomatoes from sticking, and heat over medium-low heat until the mushrooms and onion are softened.

2. Add the garlic, oregano, and basil, stir to mix, then let simmer for 5 minutes.

3. Add the cooked chicken or turkey and stir to mix. Let simmer until the chicken or turkey is heated through, about 2 minutes, then serve.

Chicken Curry

2 servings

> *Vegetable oil cooking spray (preferably canola or olive oil)*
> *1 medium onion, sliced*
> *2 teaspoons curry powder, or more to taste*
> *1 cup sliced carrots*
> *1 cup chopped celery*
> *⅔ cup uncooked basmati rice*
> *1 medium apple, chopped*
> *2 tablespoons raisins*
> *8 ounces cooked skinless, boneless chicken breast or turkey breast*
> *(page 75)*

1. Spray oil in a nonstick skillet, then place it over medium heat.

2. Add the onion and curry powder, stir to coat the onion with the curry, then sauté for 1 minute.

3. Add the carrots and celery, stir to mix, then sauté for 1 minute.

4. Add the rice, apple, raisins, and 1 cup of water, and stir to mix. Cover the skillet, reduce the heat, and let the curry simmer until all the liquid is absorbed.

5. Add the cooked chicken or turkey and stir to mix. Cook until the chicken or turkey is heated through, about 2 minutes, then serve.

Fish: Basic Preparation

1 serving

Virtually any fish is suitable, but *never* use fish that is commercially breaded or in a batter. Salmon and trout are both great favorites at our house. Pre-spiced or flavored fish is okay, but why pay someone else a whopping premium for a taste you can easily achieve yourself? Here are directions for cooking a fish fillet in a microwave oven. It couldn't be easier. Proportions are for one serving and can be multiplied as necessary.

> *1 fish fillet (4 to 5 ounces)*
> *1 to 2 teaspoons fresh lemon juice*
> *Black pepper*

1. Place the fish fillet in a microwave-safe dish.

2. Sprinkle the lemon juice and a dash of pepper over the fish.

3. Cover the dish with microwave-safe plastic wrap, folding back one corner slightly to allow the steam to escape.

4. Microwave the fish on high power until it is opaque in color and flakes when a fork is inserted, 4 to 5 minutes, rotating the dish 45 degrees halfway through cooking. Let stand for 2 minutes, then serve.

Variations

Sprinkle the fish with fresh or dried herbs, such as dill, parsley, basil, and/or tarragon.

Cook the fish on a bed of sliced leeks and onions. (Do not add oil.)

Sprinkle the fish with a mixture of whole wheat bread crumbs and chopped parsley (1 tablespoon per fillet) combined with 1 teaspoon melted light nonhydrogenated margarine.

a green light for side dishes

Need some ideas for what to serve alongside the poultry, fish, or meat? Here are a few easy-to-prepare side dishes that fit right in with the G.I. Diet.

- Green beans with almonds or mushrooms

- Mixed vegetables, such as sliced carrots, broccoli or cauliflower florets, and halved Brussels sprouts

- Boiled small, preferably new potatoes (2 to 3 per serving), tossed with chopped herbs and a smidgen of olive oil

- Basmati rice. (You can stir some extra vegetables into the rice during the last minute of cooking.) Limit the serving size to 3 tablespoons uncooked rice, which will give you ⅔ cup when cooked, covering a quarter of the plate.

- Pasta—about 1¼ ounces uncooked, for ¾ cup cooked, covering a quarter of the plate

Meat

Veal and lean deli ham are your best choices. Red meat in general is a yellow-light food, although for pragmatic reasons, I've included lean cuts of beef and extra-lean ground beef in Phase I. Pork and lamb tend to have a higher fat content and should be avoided until Phase II. The serving size is critical. Remember, use the palm of your hand or a pack of playing cards as a guide to portion size. And please do not be alarmed by the apparently modest size of these servings. I had a real problem downsizing my steak at first, but now my stomach reels at the portions served in many restaurants.

Meat Loaf

6 servings

1 ½ pounds extra-lean ground beef (less than 10 percent fat)
1 cup tomato juice
½ cup large-flake, rolled, or steel-cut oats
1 omega-3 egg, lightly beaten
½ cup chopped onion
1 tablespoon Worcestershire sauce
¼ teaspoon salt (optional)
¼ teaspoon black pepper
Steamed vegetables, for serving
12 to 18 boiled small potatoes, preferably new, for serving

1. Preheat the oven to 350°F.

2. Combine the beef, tomato juice, oats, egg, onion, Worcestershire sauce, salt, if using, and pepper in a large bowl. Mix gently but thoroughly.

3. Press the meat loaf mixture into an 8-by-4-inch loaf pan.

4. Bake the meat loaf for about 1 hour, or until an instant-read meat thermometer inserted into the center registers 160°F.

5. Let the meat loaf stand for 5 minutes before draining off any juices and slicing it. Serve the meat loaf with steamed vegetables and 2 to 3 small potatoes per person.

Variation: Extra-lean ground beef is still relatively high in fat. A lower-fat and better alternative to ground beef is an equal amount of ground turkey or chicken breast. When fully cooked, ground turkey or chicken will register 170°F on an instant-read meat thermometer.

---

steak dinner

Though strictly yellow-light, have a complete steak dinner as an occasional treat.

- Broil or grill fully trimmed steaks (4 ounces per person).

- Sauté sliced onions and mushrooms with a little water in a nonstick skillet until softened. Use the onion and mushrooms to top the steak.

- Season chopped broccoli, asparagus, and halved Brussels sprouts with nutmeg and pepper, then microwave on high until tender, about 3 to 5 minutes. (Asparagus will cook the fastest; the Brussels sprouts will require the most time.)

- Boil 3 tablespoons uncooked basmati rice or two to three small, preferably new potatoes per person. Season the cooked potatoes with chopped herbs and a touch of olive oil.

Chili

4 servings

2 teaspoons olive oil
1 large onion, sliced
2 cloves garlic, minced
½ pound extra-lean ground beef
    (less than 10 percent fat) or ground turkey
    (optional)
2 green bell peppers, chopped
2 cups canned tomatoes with juice
1 to 2 tablespoons chili powder
½ teaspoon cayenne pepper (optional)
¼ teaspoon salt
½ teaspoon chopped fresh basil
    (or ¼ teaspoon dried)
2 cups water
1 can (19 ounces) red kidney beans,
    rinsed and drained
1 can (19 ounces) white kidney beans
    (cannellini),
    rinsed and drained
Chopped tomato, chopped fresh parsley
    or cilantro, and/or yogurt cheese
    (see the box on page 84) for garnish (optional)

1. Heat the olive oil in a deep skillet or saucepan over medium heat. Add the onion and garlic and sauté until nearly tender.

2. Add the ground meat, if using, and cook until browned, breaking up the chunks with a spoon. Drain off any fat.

3. Add the bell peppers, tomatoes, chili powder, cayenne, if using, salt, basil, and water, and bring to a boil. Lower the heat and let simmer, uncovered, until the chili has reached the desired consistency, about 45 minutes.

4. Add the red and white kidney beans and cook over medium-low heat until heated through, about 5 minutes. Garnish the chili with tomato, parsley, cilantro, and/or yogurt cheese if desired. Serve.

---

yogurt cheese

Looking for a green-light alternative to sour cream? Try yogurt cheese—it's easy to make your own from plain nonfat yogurt. Place a sieve lined with cheesecloth or paper towels on top of a bowl. Spoon the yogurt into the sieve and cover it with plastic wrap. Place the sieve and bowl in the refrigerator. Let the yogurt drain overnight—the next day you'll have yogurt cheese.

SNACKS

Snacks play a critical role between meals, giving you a boost when you need it most. Have three a day: midmorning, midafternoon, and before bed. Most popular snack foods are disastrous from a sugar and fat standpoint. Commercial cookies, muffins, and candy bars should be avoided at all times. Fortunately, there are equally satisfying alternatives that are both convenient and low in cost. Never leave home without them.

On pages 86 and 87, you'll find two recipes for between-meal pick-me-ups that won't weigh you down.

---

snacking made simple

Below is a list of green-light snacks that require no preparation:

- 1 apple, pear, peach, or orange with a few almonds
- 4 ounces low-fat cottage cheese (1% or fat-free), mixed with 1 teaspoon low-sugar, double fruit preserves
- ¾ cup fat-free flavored yogurt with sweetener
- half a high-protein bar such as Balance or Zone (at least 12 to 15 grams protein per 50- to 60-gram bar)
- 8 to 10 almonds or hazelnuts

Homemade Apple Bran Muffins

Makes 12 muffins

> *Vegetable oil cooking spray*
> *¾ cup wheat bran cereal, such as All-Bran or Bran Buds*
> *1 cup skim milk*
> *⅔ cup whole wheat flour*
> *Sweetener equivalent to ⅓ cup sugar*
> *2 teaspoons baking powder*
> *½ teaspoon baking soda*
> *¼ teaspoon salt*
> *1 teaspoon ground allspice*
> *½ teaspoon ground cloves*
> *½ cup oat bran*
> *⅔ cup raisins*
> *1 large apple, peeled and cut into ¼-inch cubes*
> *1 omega-3 egg, lightly beaten*
> *2 teaspoons vegetable oil*
> *½ cup applesauce (unsweetened)*

1. Preheat the oven to 350°F. Spray a 12-cup muffin tin with vegetable oil cooking spray.

2. Mix the wheat bran and skim milk in a bowl and let stand.

3. In a large bowl, mix the flour, sweetener, baking powder, baking soda, salt, allspice, and cloves. Stir in the oat bran, raisins, and apple.

4. In a small bowl, combine the egg, oil, and applesauce. Stir, along with the wheat bran mixture, into the dry ingredients.

5. Spoon the batter into the prepared muffin tin. Bake until lightly browned, about 20 minutes. The muffins are done when a toothpick inserted into the center of one comes out clean. Keep the muffins in the freezer and microwave on high for about 30 seconds to warm.

Homemade Granola Bars

Makes 16 bars

1 ⅓ cups whole wheat flour
Sweetener equivalent to ⅓ cup sugar
2 teaspoons baking powder
¼ cup wheat bran cereal, such as All-Bran or Bran Buds
1 teaspoon ground cinnamon
1 teaspoon ground allspice
½ teaspoon ground ginger
½ teaspoon salt (optional)
1 ½ cups large-flake, rolled, or steel-cut oats
1 cup finely chopped dried apricots
½ cup shelled sunflower seeds
¾ cup applesauce (unsweetened)
½ cup apple juice (unsweetened)
3 omega-3 eggs
2 teaspoons vegetable oil

1. Preheat the oven to 400°F.

2. Line a shallow 8-by-12-inch baking dish with parchment paper.

3. Mix the flour, sweetener, baking powder, wheat bran, cinnamon, allspice, ginger, and salt, if using, in a large bowl. Stir in the oats, apricots, and sunflower seeds.

4. In a separate bowl, mix the applesauce, apple juice, eggs, and oil together, and add to the flour mixture.

5. Pour the batter into the prepared baking dish and spread it out evenly.

6. Bake until lightly browned, 15 to 20 minutes. Let cool and cut into 16 bars. Keep the bars in the freezer and microwave on high for about 30 seconds to warm.

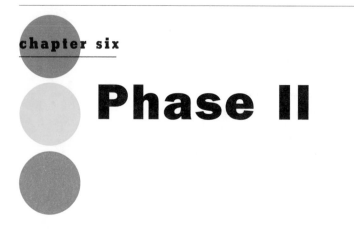

chapter six

Phase II

Congratulations! You've achieved your new target weight!

This may be hard to believe, but when I reached my target weight—I'd lost 22 pounds, and 3 inches off my waist—I had to make a conscious effort to eat more in order to avoid losing more weight. My wife said I was entering the "gaunt zone"!

PHASE II MEALS AND SNACKS

The objective in Phase II is to increase the number of calories you consume so that you maintain your new weight. Remember the equation: Food energy ingested must equal energy expended to keep weight stable. During Phase I, you were taking in less food energy than you were expending, using your fat reserves to make up the shortfall. Now we make up that deficit by taking in some extra food energy, or calories.

Two words of caution. First, your body has become accustomed to doing with fewer calories and has, to a certain extent, adapted. The result is that your body is more efficient than in the bad old days when it had more food energy than it could use. Second, your new lower weight requires fewer calories to function. For example, if you lost 10 percent of your previous weight, you'll now need 10 percent fewer calories for your body to function.

Combining a more efficient body, which requires less energy to operate, with a lower weight, which requires fewer calories, means that you need only a marginal increase in food energy to balance the energy in/energy out equation. The biggest mistake most people make when coming off a diet is assuming that they can now consume a much higher calorie level than their new body really needs. The bottom line is that Phase II is only marginally different from Phase I. Phase II provides you with an opportunity to make small adjustments to portion size and add new foods from the yellow-light category. All the fundamentals of the Phase I plan, however, remain inviolable. The following are some suggestions for how you might wish to modify your new eating pattern in Phase II:

Breakfast

- Increase cereal serving size, e.g., from ½ to ⅔ cup oatmeal.

- Add a slice of 100% whole-grain toast and a pat of margarine.

- Double up on sliced almonds on cereals.

- Help yourself to an extra slice of Canadian bacon.

- Have a glass of juice now and then.

- Add one of the forbidden fruits—a banana or apricots—to your cereal.

- Have a fully caffeinated coffee. Try to limit yourself to one a day, and make sure it's a good one!

Lunch

I suggest that you continue to eat lunch as you did in Phase I. This is the one meal that contained some compromises during the weight-loss portion of the program, since it is a meal most of us buy each day.

Dinner

- Add another boiled small new potato (from two or three to three or four).

- Increase the rice or pasta serving from ¾ cup to 1 cup.

- Have a 6-ounce steak instead of your regular 4-ounce. Make this a special treat, not a habit.

- Eat a few more olives and nuts, but watch the serving size, as these are calorie heavyweights.

- Try a cob of sweet corn with a dab of nonhydrogenated soft margarine.

- Add a slice of whole-grain rye or pumpernickel bread.

- Have a lean cut of lamb or pork (maximum 4-ounce serving).

- Have a glass of red wine with dinner.

Snacks

Warning: Strictly watch quantity or serving size.

- Light microwave popcorn (maximum 2 cups)

- Nuts, maximum eight to ten

- A square or two of bittersweet chocolate (see below)

- A banana

- One scoop of low-fat ice cream or yogurt

Chocolate

To many of us, the idea of a chocolate-free world is abhorrent. The good news is that some chocolate, in limited quantities, is acceptable.

Most chocolate contains large quantities of saturated fat and sugar, making it quite fattening. However, chocolate with a high cocoa content (70 percent or more) delivers more chocolate satisfaction per ounce. So a square or two of rich, dark, bittersweet chocolate, nibbled slowly or, better yet, dissolved in the mouth, gives us chocoholics just the fix we need. This high-cocoa chocolate is available at most supermarkets and drugstores.

Alcohol

Now is the moment that some of you have been waiting for. In Phase II, a daily glass of wine, preferably red and with dinner, is not only allowed—it's encouraged! Recently, there has been a flood of research into the benefits of alcohol on personal health. It is generally agreed that some alcohol is better than none at all, especially for heart health. As mentioned earlier, it has been found that red wine in particular is rich in flavonoids and, when drunk in moderation (a glass a day), has a demonstrable benefit in reducing the risk of heart attack and stroke. The theory that says if one glass is good for you, two must be better is tempting but not true. *One* glass provides the optimum benefit.

As with coffee, if you're going to have only one glass of wine a day, make it a great one. My eldest son took me at my word about wine and gave me a subscription to the *Wine Spectator*. It has proven to be the most costly gift I've ever received, as a whole new world of wine and wine ratings has opened up to me. My $10-a-bottle ceiling for special occasions has now doubled or tripled, though it has all been rationalized: I'm drinking less, so I can afford the extravagance!

As a beer aficionado, I like to drink the occasional beer as an alternative to wine. This habit received an endorsement from a group of scientists, who reported that beer (in moderation) would reduce cholesterol and thus heart disease, delay menopause in women, and reduce the risk of several cancers. They also noted that beer has anti-inflammatory and anti-allergic properties, plus a positive effect on bone density. Personally, I worry about any product being touted as the wonder cure for all our ills, but clearly a glass of beer with supper is likely to do little harm. But remember, because of its high malt content, beer is a high-G.I. beverage, so moderation is particularly important.

If you do drink alcohol, always have it with your meal. Food slows down the absorption of alcohol, thereby minimizing its impact.

THE WAY YOU WILL EAT FOR THE REST OF YOUR LIFE

With all these new options in Phase II, the temptation may be to overdo it. If the pounds start to reappear, simply revert to the Phase I plan for a while and you'll be astonished at how quickly your equilibrium is restored.

Phase II is the way you will eat for the rest of your life. You will look and feel better, have more energy, and experience none of those hypoglycemic lows. One reason, of course, that you have more energy is that you're not carrying around all that surplus fat. It might be fun to resurrect the water bottles and fill them up with the weight you've just lost. Carry them in shopping bags for an hour or two and then rejoice that you don't have to carry that weight for the rest of your life! Whenever your resolve wavers, reach for the water bottles. They're a marvelous motivator.

The opportunity to succeed is in your hands. I've tried to give you a simple yet motivating plan that will not leave you hungry, tired, or confused. It's all here in the book; the rest is up to you.

So head for the supermarket—and remember to park as far as possible from the entrance and enjoy the extra walk.

LIVING WITH THE G.I. DIET

One of the most popular subjects in the many e-mail messages I receive is the practicality of "living with the G.I. Diet." Let me say from the outset, although I've designed the diet to be a realistic way to eat for the rest of your life, I don't expect anyone to adhere to it 100 percent of the time. Ninety percent would be a fair average. A good illustration is the reader who told me she was on the Vegas version of the G.I. Diet and had still lost 30 pounds. Her version was to allow herself one glass of red wine a day during Phase I (acceptable in Phase II but not in Phase I). She said that without that concession, she really doubted she would have even started the diet.

"Red days," as one of my cardiologist friends calls them, are inevitable in the real world, where dining out, family celebrations, holiday meals, business travel, and vacations inevitably lend to some falling off the wagon.

Don't feel guilty when this occurs, as the worst that can happen is that it will take a little longer to realize your goals. Fortunately, one of the advantages of the G.I. Diet is the reaction of your body to red-light foods. After a few weeks of eating the G.I. Diet way, your body becomes accustomed to low-G.I. foods that keep a steady sugar level in your blood. Eat a high-G.I. red-light food and immediately your sugar level zooms and a surge of insulin kicks in, leaving a surprised body fighting to regain its equilibrium!

Some people, like our glass-of-wine-a-day reader, find they can't live without certain products. Peanut butter is another good example. If a certain food is that important to you, by all means eat it, but do so in strict moderation: for example, a 1-tablespoon serving of peanut butter per day. Otherwise, you're only kidding yourself, and risk seriously slowing your progress.

We are all faced with inevitable situations in which the menu is beyond our control: Thanksgiving, Christmas, weddings, business lunches, etc. Here are a few suggestions on how to minimize their impact on your program while still enjoying the occasion:

- Ask for extra vegetables in lieu of potatoes.

- Ask for salad dressing on the side so you control the quantity.

- Split a dessert with someone.

- Do not drink alcohol. In social situations, the pressure to drink "more than one" is very high and alcohol also tends to stimulate the appetite—a double whammy! Instead, you can choose a nonalcoholic beverage that looks like the real thing, such as sparkling soda with a slice of lemon or lime.

- Don't rush your food. It takes up to twenty minutes for your tummy to tell your brain that it's full. Also, the sooner you finish your food, the faster the opportunity and pressure for second helpings kick in.

- A detachable travel and dining-out guide is available on pages 152 to 153 for quick reference on what to eat when you have some control over the menu.

Treat Phase II as part of your reward for achieving your goals in Phase I. Don't view the G.I. Diet as overly restrictive. That is the road to certain disappointment.

An important guideline for living with the G.I. Diet is *moderation*. Although green-light products can in general be eaten in any quantity, common sense dictates that eating a jar of sugar-free applesauce or ten homemade granola bars in one sitting is not acceptable. Common sense and moderation are key ingredients in living with the G.I. Diet and should always be borne in mind when assessing portion sizes, even with green-light foods.

Finally, exercise. While exercise is not a key component during the weight-loss period in Phase I, it is an essential component in Phase II, the way you are going to eat and live for the rest of your life. For most people, simply walking thirty minutes a day (about 3 percent of your waking day) is quite sufficient. Get off the bus two stops early on your way to and from work, or park your car a mile from the office. That alone will burn up an extra pound of fat each month, giving you a little more flexibility in your diet as well as putting a spring in your step as you celebrate the new you.

to sum up

1. Don't treat the G.I. Diet as a straitjacket. Ninety percent compliance is an acceptable norm.

2. Use moderation and common sense in intepreting the diet, especially with regard to serving and portion sizes.

3. Exercise, particularly walking, is an integral part of Phase II, the way you will eat and live for the rest of your life.

Let Me Hear From You I'm most interested in your feedback on the G.I. Diet. I would particularly like to hear about your personal experience with it and any suggestions you might be willing to share. Details are on my website, www.gidiet.com.

You will also find on the website the latest updates on the diet, reader feedback, and sample recipes.

chapter seven

Eating Out

One of the most difficult challenges when trying to lose weight is eating out. You lose much of the control over content and preparation that you enjoy at home, though with a little care you can still eat the green-light way.

Dining out is more often than not a social occasion with family, friends, or coworkers, and there's a risk of fellow diners egging you on to "live a little," which usually means poor food choices, extra drinks, and inevitably, decadent desserts. The best solution is just to be up-front and solicit your companions' support by telling them that you're trying to improve your health by reducing your weight.

FAST FOOD

Though fast-food restaurants should never be your first choice, most of the leading chains have introduced menu items that are lower in fat and calories. The main caution is the amount of sodium (salt) that is often added to offset any perceived flavor loss. Remember: Salt retains liquid—which is the last thing you need when you're trying to lose weight—and raises your blood pressure. If you are not sure about salt levels, ask your server for a nutrition information sheet, which most family and fast-food restaurant chains will provide.

Here are a couple of ground rules:

1. Always eat burgers and sandwiches opened-faced, throwing away the top slice of bread or bun.

2. Use *at most* one-third of the salad dressing normally provided in a packet, as it contains far more than you would ever need and only adds unnecessary calories and salt to your meal. Choose light or vinaigrette dressings.

3. Chicken, particularly in salads, is now featured at many fast-food restaurants. Make sure you ask for grilled chicken, not crispy (fried). For example, McDonald's crispy chicken salads have more than twice the fat and 40 percent more calories than their grilled chicken salads.

4. Stay away from salad components that are not green-light (croutons, full-fat cheese, eggs, and the like). Ask your server to hold these components, or remove them yourself.

Here is a more detailed rundown of your best choices at some of the larger fast-food chains:

Subway

This chain has been a pacesetter in the fast-food industry in reducing fat and calories in their meals. Their 6-inch subs with 6 grams or less of fat, on whole wheat or honey oat bread, are your best choices. Just be careful not to load on those high-fat, high-calorie extras such as cheese, bacon, mayo, and high-sugar sauces. Low-fat (6 grams) salads are also a good choice with fat-free Italian dressing.

McDonald's

Their grilled (not crispy) chicken salads are a good bet along with one of their low-fat dressings. Grilled chicken wraps are also acceptable. You can even go for a Fruit 'n Yogurt Parfait for dessert (hold the granola).

Burger King

Their grilled chicken salads or Tendergrill Chicken Sandwich with a garden salad are your best options. You may consider the BK Veggie Burger (without mayo) and a garden salad. Remember to use only fat-free dressing. Warning: The salads are loaded with sodium—frequently more than an entire day's supply in a single meal.

Wendy's

Your best choices are the Ultimate Chicken Grill sandwich or the Grilled Chicken Go Wrap. You might also consider a large chili with a side salad. Their Mandarin Chicken and Chicken Caesar salads are fine providing you use fat-free French or balsamic vinaigrette dressing.

Pizza Hut

Normally, I recommend avoiding pizza restaurants like the plague, so I'm delighted to see that Pizza Hut has made a real effort to improve their offerings. Your best bet is their 12-inch Thin 'N Crispy Pizza (two slices maximum), plus a garden salad and light dressing.

Taco Bell

Their line of Fresco tacos and burritos are acceptable green-light choices, but the burritos have a horrendous sodium level—double that found in the tacos. Steer clear of the rest of the menu except for the side salads.

KFC

Until recently, KFC was the place to avoid. With the introduction of roasted chicken, as opposed to the traditional fried, some acceptable alternatives have opened up. Your best choices are roasted chicken salads with light dressing or the Tender Roast Sandwich and Oven Roasted Twister *without sauce*.

Quiznos

All the Turkey Subs are acceptable, plus Ham and Swiss, and Honey Bourbon Chicken. All salads (except Classic Cobb), with balsamic vinaigrette, are fine. Throw away the flatbread; it's loaded with fat and calories.

Arby's

Virtually everything they offer is loaded with fat and sodium. If you must eat here, the Chopped Turkey Club Salad or Chopped Farmhouse Chicken Salad—grilled—with a third of a pouch of balsamic vinaigrette dressing *verge* on acceptable.

Note: As fast-food menus are a dynamic field and are constantly being modified, please check individual websites from time to time to see if menus have changed.

RESTAURANTS

As it's almost impossible to list restaurants by name because of the regional nature of many chains, I thought it might be helpful to provide you with a quick rundown of green-light offerings at different types of restaurants instead.

Family Restaurants

These restaurants offer a very wide choice of foods and good value. However, the one overriding caution is portion size. Many serving sizes at these restaurants are large enough for two people. On a recent road trip, my wife and I found we could split many, if not most, of the courses and still come away satisfied. I've detailed our trip later in this chapter. If you're careful, you can easily find many green-light alternatives to suit the whole family. The Top 10 Dining Out Tips listed at the end of this chapter are particularly applicable to family restaurants.

All-You-Can-Eat Buffets

These can be your worst or best option, depending on your level of self-control. It's best to do a quick reconnaissance of the whole buffet before you start to fill your plate. This way you can pick out your best green-light choices ahead of time. Always start with a salad and a glass of water.

Italian

I suggest you begin with a good bean and vegetable soup such as minestrone. For the main course your best option is grilled, roasted, or braised fish, chicken, or veal. If you wish, you may order pasta as a side dish, but no cream sauces. You'll be better off with an extra serving of vegetables.

Greek

Grilled or baked seafood is an excellent choice, as is the classic chicken souvlaki. Just watch your serving sizes. Instead of potatoes, which are frequently served along with rice, order double vegetables. It's essential that you ask for both your salad dressing and feta to be served on the side.

Chinese

This type of food can present some real challenges. Much of it is deep-fried and comes with sweet sauces. Sodium levels are usually astronomical and the rice is glutinous and therefore red-light (short-grain rice has a much higher G.I. than long-grain rice such as basmati). Although you can make do with steamed or stir-fried vegetables, nearly everything else is loaded with temptation. A Chinese restaurant would be my last resort when eating out.

Indian/South Asian

These are two of your best restaurant choices because of the cuisines' focus on vegetables, legumes, lentils, and long-grain rice. Servings of meat, poultry, or fish tend to be modest; however, make sure that the food is not fried, particularly not in ghee (clarified butter), which is a highly saturated fat. Also be cautious with the side dishes such as mangoes, papayas, raisins, and coconut slices, as they have a higher G.I. and can pack on the calories.

Mexican/Latin American

These dishes can be heavy on cheese, refried beans, and sour cream, which are all red-light. Your best bet is to look for grilled seafood, meat, or chicken, as well as dishes made with regular, not refried, beans. Vegetable-based soups such as gazpacho are an excellent choice.

Thai

Thai restaurants tend to be heavy on red-light sauces, often using full-fat coconut milk. Here it's best to stick with a starter such as lemongrass soup, green mango salad, or mussels in lemongrass broth. Follow this with a Thai beef salad or stir-fry with chicken and vegetables. Skip the peanut sauce.

Japanese

A good green-light choice once you get beyond the sushi and tempura. Sushi is red-light because of the glutinous rice it is made with. Order the sashimi instead. Watch the quantity of soy sauce, which should be thought of as liquid salt! The beef and vegetable stir-fries and grilled fish are excellent choices. You might try nabe-mono, a healthy fondue with broth, rather than oil, as the cooking medium.

DINING AND DRIVING IN THE U.S.A.

Not long ago, my wife, Ruth, and I drove from Buffalo, New York, to Florida and back for the first time. The 3,000-plus-mile trip was part vacation—a condo rental in Naples on the Gulf Coast—and part research. We were curious to know if it was realistic, or even possible, to eat the green-light way in family-style restaurants on the road. By family-style restaurants we don't mean fast food as epitomized by McDonald's, Arby's, Burger King, and KFC, but moderately priced dine-in restaurants with large menus, such as Applebee's, Cracker Barrel, and Perkins. This is where Middle America usually dines out.

In spite of the financial recession, or perhaps because of it, these restaurants were invariably packed whenever we stopped on our way through New York State, Pennsylvania, West Virginia, the Carolinas, Georgia, and Florida. A few general observations before turning to food: First, the average customer was considerably overweight. This was not surprising, given the statistics: Over two thirds of Americans are either overweight or obese. And it was clear that children were following in their parents' footsteps.

The causes were not difficult to identify: namely, portion sizes and food choices. With regard to the former, simply stated, Ruth and I split virtually every meal between us—starters, salads, entrées, and even desserts. We simply asked for an extra plate and split the food. (I did not, however, share my occasional beer!) We never once went hungry or felt deprived. The grim fact is that serving sizes in these restaurants are seriously endangering the health of Americans. One solution would be printing calorie, fat, and sodium levels next to every meal on the menu. If people become aware of what they're eating, maybe these meals will be downsized to sensible portions.

Many restaurants had senior citizens' menus (for those 55-plus) with smaller portions. These are well worth considering from both a budget and a waistline standpoint.

Putting portion size aside, the simple fact is that you can find a healthy green-light meal on the road. Fortunately, these restaurants have huge menus. Perkins, for instance, offers a choice of 75 entrées! So shortage of choice is no excuse. But to have a fighting chance of assembling a healthy meal requires two things: 1) careful reading of the menu, and 2) some discipline and focus. Remember, they're always trying to tempt you to eat more.

With all this in mind, let's deal with each meal in turn:

Breakfast

We ate all our breakfasts at our hotels. Though there were many red-light temptations, we were able to choose from a good selection of green- or yellow-light offerings:

- instant oatmeal with hot water
- fruit yogurt—look for fat-free with sweetener
- fresh fruit/fruit salad (pick around the melon)
- whole wheat toast
- scrambled eggs
- tea/skim milk

We did *not* select pastries, pancakes, muffins, hash browns, bacon, or sausages.

Lunch

As we were driving up to 500 miles per day, we opted for light lunches so we didn't run the risk of feeling sleepy.

Salad: Our entrée was frequently a salad with grilled chicken (avoid crispy), plain shrimp, or grilled fish. We asked them to hold the cheese—which seems to appear in many, if not most, meals—and the croutons. Those giant croutons are a completely unnecessary source of calories and saturated fat. Most important, we asked for low-fat dressing—preferably balsamic vinaigrette—on the side.

Wraps/sandwiches: We avoided prepared chicken/tuna salads as they are packed with mayo. Instead, we chose plain fish, chicken, turkey, or lean ham with vegetables, and asked them to hold the potato chips, fries, and once again, cheese. One day I inadvertently forgot to request a salad in lieu of fries and the resulting mountain of greasy potatoes could easily have fed a family of four.

Dinner

We usually had a green salad or vegetable soup as a starter.

Main Course:

- *Grilled chicken/fish:* With a double helping of veggies, this was a popular choice for us.
- *Pork loin chops:* A good example of portions gone wild. The single serving consisted of *two* 6-ounce lean chops, which Ruth and I happily split between us. We added an extra vegetable.
- *Pasta:* Chicken- or seafood-based pasta in a tomato, not cream-based, sauce.

Dessert: When fresh fruit wasn't available, we opted for no-sugar-added apple or berry pie and split a serving.

Snacks

In the car we brought along water, fruit (usually picked up at our hotel breakfast!), high-protein bars (12 to 15 grams protein per 50- to 60-gram bar, minimum), and green-light muffins kept in a cooler.

Drinks

We drank a lot of water. At our daily morning coffee stop, milk—let alone skim milk—could be difficult to find. At one McDonald's we had to buy a whole carton of milk because cream was the only alternative! This wasn't a problem at any of the sit-down restaurants.

The Moral

I would be less than honest if I didn't recount one instance when we were hungry, the car was low on gas, and the only food option adjacent to the gas station was a pancake house (IHOP). In earlier years, when bringing up our children, pancakes were a family favorite. So we were determined to see how we could best handle a potentially disastrous dietary situation. Though not an ideal solution, this is how we managed:

- We split a house salad—hold the cheese.
- Ruth had two poached eggs and three pancakes with no-sugar syrup.
- I had a vegetable omelet and pancakes. Delicious!

The moral is you can eat healthfully on the road—if you split meals and choose carefully.

TOP 10 DINING OUT TIPS

If you are dining with a group, you might not have the least say as to the choice of restaurant. In that case, a little planning and some careful selections can help you over the hurdles. The following 10 tips will go a long way toward ensuring that you eat well while watching your waistline.

1. If possible, just before you go out, have a small bowl of high-fiber, green-light cold cereal (such as All-Bran) with skim milk and sweetener. I often add a couple spoonfuls of fat-free flavored yogurt. This will take the edge off your appetite and get some fiber into your digestive system, which will help reduce the G.I. of your upcoming meal.

2. Once you're seated in the restaurant, drink a glass of water. It will help you feel fuller.

3. Remember to eat slowly to allow your brain the time it needs to recognize when you are full. Put your fork down between mouthfuls and savor your meal.

4. Once the basket of rolls or bread—which you will ignore—has been passed around the table, ask the server to remove it (after you've ensured that your fellow diners have had their share, of course!). The longer it stays there, the more tempted you'll be to dig in.

5. Order a soup or salad first, and tell the server you'd like it as soon as possible. This will keep you from sitting there hungry. Go for vegetable- or bean-based soups, the chunkier the better. Avoid any that are cream-based, such as vichyssoise. For salads, the golden rule is to keep the dressing on the side. Then you can use a fraction of what the restaurant would normally pour over your greens. Avoid Caesar salads, which come pre-dressed and often pack as many calories as a burger.

6. Since you probably won't get boiled small or new potatoes, and you can't always be sure of what kind of rice is being served, ask for a double serving of vegetables instead. I have yet to find a restaurant that won't oblige.

7. Stick with low-fat cuts of meat or poultry. If necessary, you can remove the skin from chicken. Fish and shellfish are excellent choices but shouldn't be breaded or battered. Tempura is more fat and flour than filling. Remember to eat only 4 to 6 ounces (the size of a pack of cards) and leave the rest. Entrée sharing is also an option.

8. As with salad dressing, ask for any sauces or gravies to be served on the side. Avoid all those that are cream-based. Use all sauces sparingly (1 to 2 tablespoons).

9. For dessert, fresh fruit and berries—without the ice cream—are your best choices. If you're hankering for something sweet, sprinkle the fruit with sweetener from one of the packets provided for coffee or tea. Most other desserts are a dietary disaster. If a birthday cake is being passed around, share your piece with someone. A couple of forkfuls with your decaf coffee should get you off the hook with minimal dietary damage!

10. Order only decaffeinated coffee. Skim-milk decaf cappuccino is our family's favorite choice.

chapter eight

Behavior Change

Changing behaviors is arguably the most important long-term component of the G.I. Diet. I would like you to read this chapter carefully and then re-read it, because it will have a significant impact on your long-term success.

By the time we reach our thirties, most people's lifestyle patterns and personal habits are well established. Change, once so welcome in youth, is much more difficult to embrace. Over the years, you have made choices that, for better or for worse, have become deeply entrenched habits. That is why changing behaviors is so difficult as we get older. Yet changing behaviors with regard to food is fundamental to your long-term success with this program.

In this chapter we will examine some behaviors that can prove challenging to dieters. Some of you may have already modified these behaviors, but there will be other habits that, whether out of ignorance or choice, have become part of your life. I can provide you with the tools to change what you eat, but changing your food behaviors is something that only you can do. As the old adage goes, "You can lead a horse to water, but you can't make him drink!"

Here are ten important behaviors that must be addressed if you are to be successful in reaching and maintaining your weight-loss goals.

1. Skipping Breakfast

This is a very common bad habit. It is estimated that a quarter of North Americans skip breakfast, and the numbers are even worse for teenagers. A study of U.S. teens showed that only 32 percent were eating breakfast regularly.

Breakfast is the most important meal of the day. By the time people get up in the morning, most haven't eaten for ten to twelve hours. As a result, skipping breakfast will most certainly cause you to snack throughout the day to stave off hunger and flagging energy levels. And chances are that you'll reach for high-calorie, high-fat foods such as doughnuts, muffins, or cookies to give you that quick fix your body feels it needs. Chances are that at the end of the day, you'll be starving and then stuffing yourself at dinner. None of these solutions is going to help shrink your waistline—quite the reverse.

2. Not Taking Time to Eat Properly

Saying "I don't have time to eat properly" creates a breeding ground for bad habits. People who don't take the time to eat properly tend to grab a coffee and Danish on their way to work, eat a store-bought muffin midmorning to boost flagging energy levels, have a slice or two of pizza with a soft drink for lunch, snack on chocolate and cookies in the afternoon in a desperate attempt to keep their eyes open, pick up some high-fat take-out food on the way home for dinner, and finally collapse in front of the TV for the evening with a beer and a bowl of pretzels. Sound familiar?

It's easy to slip into this harmful cycle of fattening convenience food and short-term energy fixes, but you'll pay for this behavior with a growing girth and mood swings as your blood sugar rockets up and down. And in reality, the amount of time required to prepare your own healthy meals and snacks is quite modest. Fifteen minutes in the morning is all it takes to prepare and eat a healthy breakfast—often the length of time it takes to get through the line for a coffee. If you can't manage to wake up fifteen minutes earlier to squeeze in a nutritious breakfast before rushing off to work, then take along a box of green-light cereal, a carton of skim milk, and a piece of fruit. The fruit and a glass of milk take no time to prepare and make a filling, nutritious snack come midmorning. And there are always places where you can get a green-light sandwich so you don't have to resort to pizza. Eating healthfully throughout the day will ensure that you have the energy when you arrive home to prepare a quick green-light dinner in the time it would have taken to drive to the take-out joint and wait for your order.

3. Grazing

The world's best grazers are teenagers. They simply cannot resist opening the fridge every time they pass it. Their rapid growth and (hopefully) high activity levels require a constant high-calorie intake. Unfortunately, grazing is a habit that many people continue into their adult lives, when this need for a high-calorie intake has passed, with disastrous results for their waistlines and health. A few nuts here, a couple of cookies there, a tablespoon or two of peanut butter, and a few glasses of juice all look pretty harmless in themselves, but taken together, they can easily total several hundred extra calories a day! And those can add up to more than twenty pounds of additional weight in a year.

On the G.I. Diet, you should be eating three meals plus three snacks a day, which means you are eating something approximately every two hours or so during your waking hours. This will reduce your temptation to graze. One reader wrote that she couldn't believe how she could be losing weight when she always seemed to be eating. She called it green-light grazing!

4. Unconscious Eating

How often have we all begun to nibble on a bowl of chips or nuts or a box of cookies while watching TV, reading a book, or talking on the phone, and then suddenly realized that we've eaten the whole lot? Too often, I would guess.

Eating should never be a peripheral activity—it should always be the focus. Eat your meals at the table, and set aside distractions such as the TV, computer, video games, or telephone while you have your snacks. This will help you to always eat consciously and to be aware of exactly how much you're ingesting.

5. Eating Too Quickly

Dr. Johnson, the famous eighteenth-century author, is said to have asserted that food should always be chewed thirty-two times before swallowing. Though this seems rather excessive, there is an important truth here. Many of us tend to eat far too quickly. It takes twenty to thirty minutes for the stomach to let the brain know it is full. If you eat too quickly, you'll continue to eat past the point at which you've had enough. The solution, then, is to eat slowly, to allow your brain to catch up with your stomach.

That's probably just one of the reasons why Mediterranean countries have lower rates of obesity: People living there take far longer to eat their meals. In those countries, mealtimes are for family and friends, for enjoying the pleasures of food—not simply a means of tackling hunger. To ensure that you're not eating more than your appetite requires, slow down and really enjoy your meal. Put your fork down between mouthfuls. Savor the flavors and textures.

6. Not Drinking Enough

Did you know that by the time you feel thirsty you're already dehydrated? Your body's need for water is second only to its need for oxygen. Up to 70 percent of the body is composed of water, and you need about eight glasses of fluids a day to replenish your supply. Yet many of us don't take the time to drink enough, and we go through the day feeling tired and hungry, which makes us reach for food when we really should be reaching for a glass of water. Our bodies aren't hungry—they're thirsty. So always carry water with you and make sure you're drinking the recommended amount. Being properly hydrated will go a long way toward helping you control your appetite and lose weight.

7. Rewarding Exercise with Food

Another common habit is to reward yourself with food for doing some exercise. Rather than allowing the exercise to be its own reward, many feel that the extra effort deserves an additional treat, which more often than not takes the form of food or a sugary drink.

This raises a couple of issues. First, one of the great myths about weight loss is that it can be achieved through exercise. *Although exercise is essential for long-term health and weight maintenance, it is actually a poor tool for losing weight.* To lose just one pound of fat, a 160-pound person would have to walk briskly for 42 miles. That is a huge amount of effort and way beyond what most people have the physical capability or time to do. Walking around the block or washing the car consumes only a handful of calories. So if you're using exercise as permission to cut a little slack in your diet, remember: That cookie reward might add more calories than you expended during your activity. By all means, exercise to improve your health and help lower your blood sugar levels, but don't think it will significantly contribute to your weight loss. I frequently tell people that losing weight is 90 percent diet and 10 percent exercise, particularly in the early stages.

8. Cleaning the Plate

From the time we were small, many of us were taught to finish the food on our plate before leaving the table. This becomes a deeply entrenched habit that does not, unfortunately, help us to lose or maintain weight later in life. Not only do we finish our own plate, but we tend to also finish the leftovers on our children's plates or that last lonely slice of pie. I confess that I did this. But this habit causes us to eat more than we need to satisfy our hunger, and is therefore dreadful for weight control. Get into the habit of letting your stomach and your brain—not the quantity of food on your plate—determine when you are full. Put out only enough food for the meal—no extras. Store leftovers in the fridge, rather than around your waist or hips.

9. Shopping on an Empty Stomach

Human nature can often be perverse, encouraging us to do the right thing but at the wrong time. When you are full and satisfied, food shopping is rarely at the top of your mind. But when you're hungry, grocery shopping suddenly seems like a very good idea indeed. Unfortunately, it just isn't: You'll end up with a shopping cart that has been filled primarily by your stomach rather than your head. Those red-light foods will seem far more tempting than usual, and you'll probably make some poor choices as a result. So always shop after a meal, or at least take a green-light snack such as an apple or half a high-protein bar with you. You'll make far wiser choices this way.

10. Eating High-Sugar, High-Fat Treats

As we are only too aware, food is a huge part of holidays and get-togethers—just picture the special foods that go along with every big occasion. And where would the candy industry be without Valentine's Day or Halloween? Food is also linked with our most intimate positive experiences, and that's another reason we often think of certain foods as treats. Whether it's Grandma doling out candies when we've been good, or a neighbor presenting us with a fresh-baked pie in gratitude for raking her leaves, we associate food with reward—for the people in our lives as well as for ourselves. Unfortunately, these so-called treats tend to be high in calories, sugar, and fat, and they are not our friends. They are a major contributor to the obesity crisis and to weight-related diseases such as diabetes and heart disease. We should really start to view these foods as penalties rather than rewards.

You can choose treats that are lower in calories and fat. If chocolate is your thing, indulge in the occasional square of high cocoa (70%) dark chocolate. Fresh fruit, fat-free yogurt with sweetener, and low-fat frozen yogurt are even better treats. And there are many delicious green-light dessert and snack recipes in all the G.I. Diet books. So don't be afraid to treat yourself every now and then—just make sure you pick the right sort of treats.

Keep in mind that although changing bad habits can be challenging at times, before you know it, your new habits will be as firmly entrenched as the old ones used to be. And these habits will help you slim down to a brand-new you.

EMOTIONAL EATING

One of the most difficult and destructive behaviors is emotional eating, wherein people seek comfort in food. I have asked my wife, Dr. Ruth Gallop, to write this section. As a professor emeritus at the University of Toronto, one of her specialties is childhood trauma and how it plays out in adult life. This has given her considerable insight into the role food plays in helping people deal with their emotional issues. We realize that this is a very broad topic, and though we can't cover every aspect of it here, we hope to provide you with some guidance. Here are some of her thoughts:

We all eat for comfort. When we are sick, many of us have favorite foods—often foods from our childhood—that we associate with being looked after. This is why certain foods can make us feel emotionally comforted and happy.

When our lives are reasonably balanced, food plays an important, but not dominant, role in our day-to-day routines. When we don't feel good about certain aspects of our lives, food can take over. If we don't have a positive self-image and consequently experience low self-esteem, food can be a powerful and damaging force. This is particularly true for women, because society is fixated on how they should look. Putting aside all the health benefits of being at a "normal" weight, our society just doesn't approve of overweight people. And more significantly, overweight people often don't approve of themselves.

Frequently, having negative feelings leads us to eat to feel better. For some people, these negative feelings may include sadness, loneliness, or boredom. For others, the feelings may be more along the lines of anger, irritability, or high stress. These feelings can lead to a vicious eating cycle that goes something like this:

> I feel depressed, angry, bored, sad, bad about myself (low self-esteem) → so I eat to feel better. → I experience a brief blood sugar high and I do feel better. → I experience a blood sugar crash and I feel terrible. → I feel bad about myself for having eaten (for failing) → so I eat to feel better . . . and around I go.

Sometimes the reasons for feeling bad about oneself—or feeling angry, overwhelmed, or disappointed—may have their origins in childhood. Overeating, negative body image, and low self-esteem are the consequences. Usually, we don't make any conscious link between past events and present behavior. When we were children, for example, parental love or approval may have been connected with food via treats or eating all that was put in front of us. Or we may have been punished (love withdrawn) if we didn't eat our vegetables! As a consequence of these childhood experiences, eating has become connected to trying to recapture the feeling of being loved. Although we may not be aware of these motives or other psychological reasons for our behavior, they have become part of our food and eating habits.

Rick's mother cannot bear to see uneaten food on the table, regardless of whether or not a person is still hungry. At ninety-nine years of age, she still says "I do like to see a clean plate" when all the food on the table has disappeared. When Rick was a child, he earned his mother's love and approval by eating all that was put in front of him. I have learned to deal with Rick's consequent learned behavior—cleaning his plate—by never putting extra food on the table at mealtimes. Instead, I make up the dinner plates before I serve them. I never put out bowls of food for helping ourselves. Otherwise, Rick would unconsciously graze through a lot of extra food!

If you are ready to change your eating habits, the first thing you need to do is become aware of them. Every time you walk in the front door, is your first stop the fridge or cookie jar? When you have had a bad day, do you deal with it by eating something sweet or creamy? When you feel bored, is eating the first activity you turn to? Are you unable to watch TV without food in your hand, so that you unconsciously end up eating more than you realize? I know I sometimes do! I have a single piece of dark chocolate most evenings if I'm watching TV. The other night I realized that I was in the middle of eating a second piece—with no memory of reaching down and picking it up!

It is important to recognize risky situations. Take a day or two to jot down your patterns and work out when automatic behaviors take over and when it's most difficult for you to avoid eating in excess. Some of these habits may include:

- Grazing.

- Eating when you're stressed, angry, irritable, tired, frustrated, sad, bored, or lonely.

- Eating too fast. Remember, it takes twenty to thirty minutes for the stomach to let the brain know it is full.

- Eating unconsciously, especially in front of the TV or at the movies.

- Eating portions that are far too large. Thanks to fast-food chains and countless restaurants, many portion sizes have doubled. Unfortunately, we have brought this portion distortion into our homes.

- Keeping red-light snacks in your desk drawer to eat when you are stressed at work.

- Eating during any social activity, whether it's a sporting event, a social visit, or even just walking with a friend.

A friend of ours, who is struggling to break poor food habits, uses a trick that you might find helpful in your efforts to do the same. He wears a plastic bracelet on his left wrist. When he makes a wrong choice he switches the bracelet to his right wrist. This reminds him every time he reaches for something to eat that he has already made one poor choice that day. (If you decide to try this, log on to www.gidiet.com and let us know how it goes!)

Once you're aware of how comfort eating plays a role in your life, you can begin to change your behavior. The first step is to make sure that all the food in your home and workplace, as well as all the food going into your mouth, is green-light. Make sure you reward yourself for this accomplishment, perhaps by going to a movie, sleeping in late, or having breakfast in bed. Indulge in a little luxury that you wouldn't normally allow yourself. Rick's idea of a treat is a trip to Home Depot! Just make sure you don't reward yourself with red-light food.

Start by trying to modify one behavior at a time. If you're in the habit of walking in the front door and immediately eating a snack, make sure you have a green-light snack at the ready. It's particularly important to have snacks with a good, sweet mouthfeel when sugar cravings take over. High-fiber fruit muffins (with raspberries, blueberries, strawberries, or peaches) make an excellent sweet snack, as do fresh berries sweetened with Splenda and perhaps a dollop of Splenda-sweetened fat-free sour cream. As the diet progresses, sugar cravings and irritability will lessen, as long as you stick with green-light foods and eat three meals and three snacks a day.

It's important to keep your hands busy as you break the habit of unconsciously grazing while you watch TV. I read books or magazines. Rick checks his e-mail. You might take up a new hobby—knitting and scrapbooking have become trendy. Or Twitter away!

Substituting pleasurable activities is an important tool for breaking bad eating habits, because if the substitute behaviors weren't enjoyable, we'd be much less likely to stick with them. Before long, your new behaviors and eating patterns will be your new habits. Don't beat yourself up if you slip—it happens to all of us. Just get back on the wagon. Having the determination to pursue this program takes courage—pat yourself on the back and get on with the journey.

It may also be helpful to think about your long-term goals. Have you always dreamed of taking up a new hobby or sport? Perhaps you've wanted to take dance lessons or learn to ski but avoided those activities because of a lack of self-esteem or poor body image. Maybe now's the time to say "This is possible." Keep that goal in your mind when you reach for a red-light food. How will it help you get out on the dance floor?

As you lose weight, you'll feel better, not only physically but psychologically, too. As you start to experience success in weight reduction—and we're talking here about permanent weight reduction—you'll start to experience yourself as successful. Successful people hold themselves differently and interact with people differently. You'll find that being successful will improve your self-esteem, and that feeling better about how you look is the best reinforcement for avoiding red-light foods and breaking those bad eating habits. Not only will you notice your body changing, but soon others will notice, too. Let people compliment you. As one reader wrote, "I no longer hide behind a tree every time a camera comes out." You'll find that a more confident "you" may feel safe enough to come out into the world.

Again, I encourage you to build in a reward for each week of success on the program—go to a show or a ballgame, buy some flowers, or take a long, luxurious bath. Don't buy the new wardrobe yet—that's for later. Just remember: Be good to yourself.

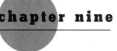
Staying Motivated

You wouldn't be human if you didn't feel your resolve starting to waver from time to time. It frequently has nothing to do with your diet but is related to family, work, or other unrelated health stressors in your life. It can be difficult to maintain your motivation during times when you feel you are not making enough progress or when your stress levels become overwhelming. When they do, however, there are a number of things you can do to encourage yourself to keep going. Here is a summary of seven of the best motivators I've come across.

1. Body Image

You want to look better. Weight loss boosts self-esteem and confidence, which in turn makes it easier to maintain your new eating habits. It's amazing the difference the loss of just a few pounds can make, not only in how you look in your clothes, but also in how you feel about yourself.

2. Energy

Although body image does not appear to be a primary motivator for men to lose weight, increased physical capability, strength, and energy can be. Most of us don't realize how much weight actually weighs. Being overweight means you have more pounds to carry around, which translates into flagging energy levels; a sore back, hips, and knees; and decreased mobility.

3. Health

What you weigh and what you eat impacts your risk of heart disease, stroke, diabetes, and most cancers. Eating the right foods can improve your health and increase your energy levels to help you lead a longer and more active life. It's hard to find a better motivator than that. Keep reminding yourself that good health is the most important asset in life and staying with this program is your best chance to promote it.

4. Physical Reminders

Judging by the number of e-mails I receive from readers about digging out "skinny" tops and pants that they had tucked away at the back of the closet, never expecting them to see the light of day again, dropping sizes is a tremendous motivator, especially for women. Most women would prefer to shop for clothes that flatter and show off their bodies rather than resort to camouflage. It's a powerful motivator to walk into a room and hear a friend ask, "Have you lost weight? You look terrific." I've sold more books based on word-of-mouth exchanges like this one than on any other marketing strategy.

Try keeping a picture of an outfit you're going to buy when you reach your goal, or a photograph of a thinner you, where you'll see it every day.

5. Your Achievements

Compare yourself now to where you were when you started the diet. How much weight have you lost? How many inches have dropped from around your waist? Add in your new energy and the clothes you've bought and you'll be amazed to see how far you've come. Going back to your old eating habits won't seem so tempting when you think of how it will undermine all the good things that this new way of living has brought you so far.

6. The Shopping Bag Motivator

As I mentioned, people frequently don't realize how much weight actually weighs. I know it sounds crazy, but when people tell me they've lost only 20 pounds, I ask them to fill plastic bottles with water until the bottles weigh 20 pounds, put them in shopping bags, and carry them up and down the stairs a few times. Everyone is always glad to put the bags down and reports that he or she had no idea how heavy 20 pounds really is.

One reader, Kathy, decided to try this test using 20-pound sacks of potatoes instead of water bottles. She wrote, "I picked up two of these, and just picking them up, they were so heavy. I thought, 'Wow, I carried all that around with me every day.' I tried to walk with them and I got tired after only about fifteen steps." Kathy decided that it wasn't worth it to put her body through so much strain. She concluded, "I like my lighter body and I'm going to keep working on it to keep it this way."

7. Get Support

Buddy up with friends, your partner, or family members who are also trying to lose weight. They will give you a sense of camaraderie and encouragement as you strive for your goal, and you can turn to them for support when you need it.

"Nothing succeeds like success" may be a cliché, but as a motivator it is second to none. Keep a tally of your successes and always keep them in front of you, especially during those times when the spirit weakens—as it inevitably will. A weight-loss graph is an excellent visual for keeping track of how far you've come.

There are a couple of occasions when motivation becomes especially crucial; namely, when you hit a weight-loss plateau or when you "fall off the wagon." Here are some suggestions for dealing with these two inevitable challenges.

REACHING A PLATEAU

After diligently eating the green-light way and losing weight steadily for successive weeks, it's difficult to accept a break in that pattern. Unfair as it may be, it's bound to happen. Weight loss never occurs in a straight line, but always in a series of steps and plateaus.

There are a couple of principal causes. For women, hormonal shifts triggered by your monthly cycle or by menopause cause the body to retain fluid. You'll know you're retaining fluid if you usually wear rings—they'll feel tight on your fingers. This is nearly always a temporary state. As your hormones shift back to their previous levels, so will your fluids.

For men and women alike, the other most common cause is "portion creep": when you have let your guard down and allowed your portions or serving sizes to increase. This slip-up is an easy one to make. You watched the pounds steadily drop off, and now, not surprisingly, complacency sets in.

A useful tool in keeping yourself on track is to divide your plate into three sections (see the diagram on page 156). Half the plate should consist of at least two vegetables; one quarter should consist of a protein (meat, fish, or tofu); and the remaining quarter can consist of rice, potatoes, or pasta. And remember to use smaller lunch-size plates instead of oversize dinner plates.

Since hormonal shifts and complacency can cause your weight to fluctuate significantly from day to day, I suggest you restrict your weigh-in to once a week, or even once a month. Then you can avoid the disappointment of short-term aberrations and focus on your long-term success. One reader wrote to me and said that she had become very frustrated with the daily variations in her weight and decided to weigh herself once a month. She said that there had not been a single month in the past eighteen in which she had not lost some weight, and her frustration level had dropped significantly.

When playing the averages, patience is a virtue! Just keep on the green-light track and the weight will continue to come off. Some readers wonder why they sometimes seem to be losing inches but not pounds, and sometimes pounds but not inches. Remember, everyone is different, and weight loss doesn't ever happen in a straight line; eventually both the inches and pounds will come off—guaranteed!

So don't let a disappointment on the scale get you down. If you hang in there and don't use food to console yourself, you will reach your weight-loss target.

FALLING OFF THE WAGON

Like a weight-loss plateau, falling off the wagon is inevitable. And while I don't encourage it, it's acceptable as long as it's the exception and not the rule. The G.I. Diet isn't written in stone. If you do your best to eat the green-light way 90 percent of the time, you will still lose weight. The odd lapse will, at worst, delay you from reaching your target weight by a week or two. So don't be too hard on yourself, and just get right back on the plan at the next meal. Some people make the mistake of feeling so badly about slipping up that they just give up. But you should anticipate that you will fall off the wagon from time to time. The best way to handle this is to learn why it happened and decide how you'll handle the situation next time. By now you have the knowledge and tools to do just that.

Although most people find that their cravings diminish after a few weeks on the G.I. Diet (because of the leveling effect green-light eating has on blood sugar levels), there will be times when a craving will hit. Following are some suggestions for how to handle these situation.

1. Try to distract yourself with an activity. Call a friend, fold a basket of laundry, check your e-mail, read a book, or just go for a walk. Frequently, a craving will pass.

2. If you still have the craving, pinpoint the flavor that you want and find a green-light food that has it. For example, if you want something sweet and creamy, try fat-free yogurt or low-fat ice cream with no added sugar. If you want something salty, have a couple of olives or a dill pickle, or some hummus with veggies. If it's chocolate you crave, try half a chocolate-flavored high-protein bar or a mug of instant light hot chocolate. There are many green-light versions of the foods we normally reach for when a craving strikes.

3. Sometimes nothing but a piece of chocolate or a spoonful of peanut butter will do. If this is the case, have a *small* portion and really enjoy it. Eat it slowly and savor the experience. Chalk it up to that 10 percent leeway you're allowed on the G.I Diet. Just make sure you're staying green-light 90 percent of the time. This 10 percent "wiggle room" gives you permission to enjoy that extra serving or occasional drink. It is meant to help you stay with the program, so use it wisely!

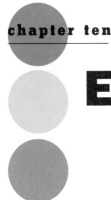

chapter ten

Exercise

Earlier in the book, I suggested that weight loss was 90 percent diet and 10 percent exercise, even though exercise is essential for weight maintenance and a healthy lifestyle. To recap, there are two principal reasons why exercise is not as efficient as diet when you are trying to lose weight. First, it requires a huge amount of effort to burn off those pounds, and second, it takes a great deal of time. Take a good look at the table below.

EFFORT REQUIRED TO LOSE 1 POUND OF FAT

	130-pound person	160-pound person
Walking (briskly—4 mph)	53 miles/13¼ hrs	42 miles/10½ hrs
Running (8-minute mile)	36 miles/4½ hrs	29 miles/3½ hrs
Cycling (12–14 mph)	96 miles/7–8 hrs	79 miles/6–7 hrs
Sex (average effort)	79 times	64 times

I'm sure many of you have tried working out on a treadmill or an exercise bike at some time in your life and have been amazed at how much effort it takes to burn even 200 calories. As one pound of fat contains 3,600 calories, you can see why taking the dog for a walk around the block or washing the car has little or no impact on losing weight. Obviously, any exercise is better than none, as it all helps to burn extra calories. Just don't expect it to have any significant impact during the weight-loss phase.

However, if you are nearing your weight-loss goals, this is the time to consider being more active. The upside of exercise is that, *over the long term,* it can help you maintain or accelerate your weight loss; plus it contributes significantly to your health by reducing your risk of heart disease, stroke, diabetes, and osteoporosis. It will also help maintain your muscle mass and tone.

Exercise should become an important consideration for anyone moving from being "obese" to being "overweight." You should be better able to exercise now that you're experiencing an increase in your energy levels. I believe that when you have your diet under control, fewer pounds to carry around, and more energy, it's time to get more active.

The simplest activity is walking. This doesn't require any special equipment or gym membership, and can be done at virtually any time of the day or year. Walking thirty minutes a day, seven days a week, should be your target. If you add an hour-long walk on the weekend, you can take a day off during the week. I'm talking about brisk walking—not speed walking, not ambling. It must increase your heart and breathing rate, but you should never exercise to the point at which you cannot find the breath to converse with a partner.

You don't need any special clothing or equipment except a comfortable pair of sneakers. And walking is rarely boring, since you can keep changing routes and watch the world go by while you exercise. Walk with a friend for company and mutual support, or go solo and commune with nature and your own thoughts. I do my best thinking of the day on my morning walk. This is not surprising when you realize how much extra oxygen-fresh blood is pumping through your brain.

A great idea is to incorporate walking into your daily commute to work. For instance, get off the bus two stops early and walk the rest of the way. If you drive to work, try parking your car a mile or so away and walking to your job. You may even find cheaper parking farther out. This investment of an extra 10 or 15 minutes a day each way will pay real dividends for maintaining your weight and health.

I used to do this and found that, far from being a "drag" or an inconvenience, I actually looked forward to my "two stops short" walk each day. It helped get me going in the morning and gave me time to prepare for my day with no phones ringing or people crowding me. In the evening, it provided me with a chance to wind down and relax. Getting started required some effort during the first week, but my daily walks quickly became a routine part of my last three years at the Heart and Stroke Foundation.

By now, many of you will be muttering about how this would all sound fine if we lived in California, but many of us have either frigid, snowy winters or hot, humid summers to contend with, making outdoor activities unappealing. The alternative is either a home gym or a health club. The latter is an easy option these days in most larger communities. Clubs offer not only a wide range of sophisticated equipment, but also mutual support from other members and expert advice from staff. If possible, have a trainer develop a program for you and show you how to use the equipment properly.

If a health club isn't convenient, if membership is too expensive, or if those Lycra-clad young things make you uncomfortable, the simple alternative is to exercise at home. The best and least expensive equipment is a stationary exercise bike.

You can easily pay into the thousands for a stationary bike with all the fancy trimmings, designed for use in a health club, but in reality the $200 to $300 machine will work fine. Just be sure it has smooth, adjustable tension and a proper seat height, then put on a DVD or your favorite soap opera and get pedaling. You'll be amazed how quickly the minutes fly by. I've frequently gone way over my scheduled time as I've become immersed in the onscreen action! Twenty minutes on the bike will result in the same calorie consumption as thirty minutes of brisk walking.

The recumbent bikes (in which you sit against a backrest, with your legs out in front) are probably easier on your joints, as your weight is spread over a greater area. These are also relatively inexpensive and available through many large retail chains.

If biking is not for you, try a treadmill. These can be expensive—expect to pay about $700 to $1,000. Beware the lower-end models that cannot take the pounding, and make sure the incline of the track can be raised and lowered for a better workout.

In summary, aerobic exercise is of somewhat limited value during the period when you are actually losing weight. It is, however, a critical factor in maintaining your weight and health for the rest of your life. Believe it or not, exercise can become addictive—I know that I become irritable and edgy if I don't get my daily workout, or so my wife tells me!

So far, I have focused on aerobic exercise—the sort that increases your heart rate—but there are several other types of exercise you should think about. The most important of these are resistance exercises, which are aimed at strengthening your muscles.

An insidious and silent change that takes place as we age is the loss or thinning of muscle mass. This is a process that starts in our twenties, and by middle age most people have already lost around 15 percent of their muscle mass. From middle age onward, the rate of muscle loss escalates quickly. So why does this loss matter? First, you risk becoming frail, as you lack muscle to move and stabilize your body. Without strong muscles in your legs and hips, women in particular are at significant risk of a debilitating fall, broken bones, or worse.

Second, less muscle means a lower metabolic rate. Muscles are the principal consumer of your body's energy (calories); so the less muscle, the fewer calories you burn—and we all know where those surplus calories go. Fat replaces muscle, and fat burns few calories.

However, all is not lost. There are a couple of things you can do to help offset this decline and raise your metabolic rate.

The first is to make sure you are getting adequate protein in your diet. The best sources of lean protein are chicken and turkey (skinless), fish, eggs (liquid), lean red meats, low-fat dairy, soy, and legumes (beans). Ideally, every snack and certainly every meal should have some protein content. A further benefit of protein is that it slows digestion and therefore effectively lowers the G.I. of the meal.

The second offset is resistance exercise. When exercised in this manner, muscles work against some form of resistance; weights and elastic bands are the two most popular forms. These are the only exercises that build muscle mass. I'm sure many of you associate weights with an image of overly muscled men sweating and grunting with giant barbells. The reality is far less daunting— even a can of soup can act as a weight.

I won't detail a specific program here, as everyone's needs and budgets are different. Rather, I recommend going to the Physical Activity page of the U.S. Government's Centers for Disease Control and Prevention website (www.cdc.gov/physicalactivity) and clicking on "Growing Stronger—Strength Training for Older Adults." On that page, click on "Exercises." This is an excellent site that demonstrates how to do the various exercises—and it's free!

Boosting your protein intake and adding a few minutes of simple resistance exercises three times a week will go a long way toward stabilizing your muscle loss and, if you are diligent, actually rebuilding some of that loss. You will be less frail and less prone to falling, and you will burn more calories. Remember, muscles consume calories even when they are at rest and even when you're sleeping.

GETTING STARTED

Once you've decided that exercise is for you, just how do you go about getting started?

1. Select a workout that suits you. The fastest way to abandon an exercise program is to do something you don't enjoy. It is best to select an exercise that uses the largest muscle groups—that is, the legs, abdominals, and lower back. These burn more calories because of their sheer size. Walking and biking are excellent choices.

2. Check with your doctor to ensure that he or she supports your plan.

3. Set goals and keep a record of your progress. Put the log on the fridge or in the bathroom.

4. Get support from family and friends. If possible, find a like-minded buddy to exercise with you.

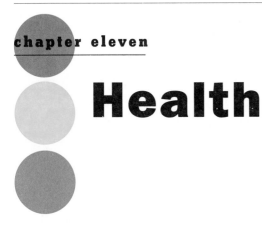

chapter eleven

Health

Foods impact our health in two ways. First, your choice of foods and the quantity you consume are key determinants in how much you weigh. And the connection between being overweight and an increased risk for diseases such as heart disease, stroke, and diabetes is well established.

Second, the types of protein, fat, and carbohydrates you consume can determine your risk level for heart disease, stroke, diabetes, prostate and colon cancers, and Alzheimer's disease.

Foods are, in effect, drugs. They have a powerful influence on our health, well-being, and emotional state. And we take in food four or five times a day, usually with more thought for taste than for nutritional value.

The right foods can help you maintain your health, extend your life span, give you more energy, and make you feel good and sleep better. Couple that with exercise and you are doing all you can to keep healthy, fit, and alert. The rest is a matter of genes and luck.

Making the right choices has been the principal theme of the G.I. Diet. We'll now examine the role of diet and exercise in preventing diseases and providing you with all the nutrients necessary for a healthy life.

HEART DISEASE AND STROKE

Given that I was the president of the Heart and Stroke Foundation of Ontario for fifteen years, it is hardly surprising that I'm starting with a discussion of these diseases. However, there is a more important reason: Heart disease and stroke cause 35 percent of North American deaths. Remarkably, this is evidence of progress. When I first joined the foundation, the figure was close to 50 percent.

This is a good news/bad news story. The good news is that advances in surgery, drug therapies, and emergency services have saved many lives. The bad news is that twice as many deaths could have been averted if only we had reduced our weight, exercised regularly, and quit smoking. Though the smoking rate for adults has dropped sharply (unfortunately, we cannot say the same for teens), we are eating more and exercising less, leading inevitably to a more obese and unhealthy population. It's been calculated that if we led even moderate lifestyles, we could halve the carnage from these diseases. Although heart disease, like most cancers, is primarily a disease of old age, nearly half of those who suffer heart attacks are under the age of sixty-five.

A familiar refrain I hear is, "Why worry? If I have a heart attack, modern medicine will save me." It might well save you from immediate death, but what most people don't realize is that the heart is permanently damaged after an attack. The heart cannot repair itself because its cells don't reproduce. (Ever wonder why you can't get cancer of the heart? That's the reason.) After the damage sustained during a heart attack, the heart has to work harder to compensate—but it rarely can. So make sure you do everything you can to avoid a heart attack in the first place.

For many years, heart attacks were considered to be a man's domain. More often than not, this is still the case for people under the age of 50; however, for men *and* for women aged 50-plus, it becomes a shared risk. With regard to diet, the simple fact is that the more overweight you are, the more likely it is that you will suffer a heart attack or stroke. The two key factors linking heart disease and stroke to diet are high cholesterol and hypertension (high blood pressure). I promised at the beginning of this book that I was not going to dwell on the complexities of the science of nutrition; it's the outcome of this science that's important. However, a little science is helpful to understand the role and significance of both hypertension and cholesterol.

Hypertension is the harbinger of both heart disease and stroke. High blood pressure puts more stress on the arterial system and causes it to age and deteriorate more rapidly, ultimately leading to arterial damage, blood clots, and heart attack or stroke. Excess weight has a major bearing on high blood pressure. Recent research has shown that a lower-fat diet coupled with a major increase in fruits and vegetables (eight to ten servings a day) lowered blood pressure. The moral: Lose weight and eat more fruits and vegetables to help reduce your blood pressure levels. In other words, adopt the G.I. Diet.

Cholesterol is essential to your body's metabolism. High cholesterol, however, is a problem, as it's the key ingredient in the plaque that can build up in your arteries, eventually cutting off the blood supply to your heart (causing a heart attack) or your brain (leading to stroke). To make things more complicated, there are two forms of cholesterol: HDL (good) cholesterol and LDL (bad) cholesterol. The idea is to boost the HDL level while depressing the LDL level. (Remember it this way: HDL is Heart's Delight Level and LDL is Leads to Death Level.)

The villain that raises LDL levels is saturated fat, which is usually solid at room temperature and is found primarily in meat and whole milk and certain other food products. Conversely, polyunsaturated and monounsaturated fats not only lower LDL levels but actually boost HDL. The moral: Make sure some fat is included in your diet, but make sure it's the right fat. (Refer to chapter 1, The Problem, for the complete rundown on fat.)

DIABETES

Diabetes is the kissing cousin of heart disease, in the sense that more people die from heart complications arising from diabetes than from diabetes alone. And diabetes rates are skyrocketing: They're expected to double in the next ten years.

The principal causes of the most common form of diabetes, type 2, are obesity and lack of exercise, and the current epidemic is strongly correlated to the obesity trend.

Foods with a low G.I., which release sugar more slowly into the bloodstream, appear to play a major role in helping diabetics control their disease. Thus the G.I. Diet provides an opportunity both to lose excess weight and to assist in the management of the symptoms.

Because protein and fat have an impact on food's G.I. ratings, diabetics should be particularly careful about eating the right balance of green-light proteins, carbohydrates, and fats at every meal and snack. Prevention, however, is far preferable, so get right into your G.I. Diet program and exercise plan, and get those pounds off.

CANCER

In one of the largest studies on obesity and cancer to date, British scientists pooled information from 141 studies on 20 different cancers. They found conclusive evidence that obesity is replacing smoking as the number one risk factor for cancer. They demonstrated a depressing series of linkages between being overweight and several types of cancers:

- Thyroid, kidney, and colon cancers; cancer of the esophagus; multiple myeloma; leukemia; and non-Hodgkin's lymphoma in both sexes.

- Rectal cancer and malignant melanoma in men.

- Gallbladder, pancreatic, endometrial, and postmenopausal breast cancer in women.

In addition, a global report by the American Institute for Cancer Research concluded that 30 to 40 percent of cancers are directly linked to dietary choices. Its key recommendation is that individuals should choose a predominantly plant-based diet that includes a variety of vegetables, fruits, and grains and is low in saturated fat—the G.I. Diet in a nutshell.

ALZHEIMER'S DISEASE

As with cancer, there is increasing evidence linking certain dementias, particularly Alzheimer's, with fat intake. A recent U.S. study showed a 40 percent higher rate of Alzheimer's disease in people who ate a diet high in saturated fat.

ABDOMINAL FAT AND HEALTH

The most alarming medical news about fat is that it is not, as previously thought, a passive accumulator of energy reserves and extra baggage. Rather it is an active, living part of your body. Once it has formed sufficient mass, it behaves like any other organ, such as the liver, heart, or kidney, except that it pumps out a dangerous combination of free fatty acids and proteins. This causes out-of-control cell proliferation, which is directly associated with the growth of malignant cancer tumors. It also creates inflammation, which is linked to atherosclerosis (hardening of the arteries), the principal cause of heart disease and stroke. And if that weren't bad enough, fat tissues also increase insulin resistance, leading to type 2 diabetes.

The fact is that abdominal fat has many of the characteristics of a huge tumor—and that thought may help encourage any fence-sitters out there to start doing something about their weight.

KNEE AND HIP REPLACEMENT

Finally, there is the issue of joint degeneration caused by excessive weight. A survey of knee and hip replacements performed in Canada in 2004 and 2005 showed that not only had the number of operations nearly doubled over the past ten years, but overweight and obese patients accounted for a startling 87 percent of knee replacements and 74 percent of hip replacements. Interestingly, 60 percent of patients were women, whose smaller bone structure makes them more vulnerable to extra weight stress.

The U.S. has recorded similar figures, with a 48 percent increase in hip and 63 percent increase in knee operations between 1997 and 2004.

So if you want to reduce your risk of incurring these leading killer diseases—heart disease, stroke, diabetes, hypertension, and cancer—and keep your joints intact, then stay with the program. I can't think of a better motivator.

SUPPLEMENTS

Provided you're eating the green-light way, you are receiving all the nutrients you need for a healthy life. There are, however, two important exceptions:

Vitamin D

Vitamin D is known as the "sunshine vitamin" for very good reason. It is generated by the action of sunlight on our skin. Found in food only in very limited quantities, it's primarily confined to fatty fish, such as salmon, or fortified milk products. This vitamin is particularly important in reducing your risk for diabetes, cancer, heart disease, and osteoporosis. The problem is that for those of us in northern climates, sunshine is a scarce commodity in winter, and since we should be lathered in sunscreen during our summers, we are unable to capitalize on this vitamin self-generation. Most authorities now recommend a daily supplement of 1,000 milligrams of this inexpensive vitamin.

Fish Oil

There is one oil in particular that has been found to have significant health benefits, especially for your heart. The oil, called omega-3, is a fatty acid found primarily in coldwater fish—salmon in particular—and in modest amounts in canola and flaxseed. As most of us are unlikely to consume enough salmon, or canola or flaxseed on a daily basis, consider taking salmon oil, available in capsule form in any pharmacy.

---

to sum up

The G.I. Diet almost certainly contains sufficient vitamins to meet your daily needs. However, if you are at all concerned, a one-a-day multivitamin offers cheap and risk-free insurance. An extra vitamin D pill is an excellent idea, particularly if you live in the north, but keep your ears and eyes open to new research on this front. If heart health is a particular concern, omega-3 oil capsules are a good idea.

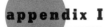

The Complete G.I. Diet Food Guide

	RED LIGHT	YELLOW LIGHT	GREEN LIGHT
beans/peas	Baked beans with pork		Baked beans (low-fat, ½ cup)
	Fava beans		Black beans
	Refried beans		Black-eyed peas
			Butter beans
			Cannellini
			Chickpeas (garbanzo beans)
			Haricot beans
			Italian beans
			Kidney beans
			Lentils
			Lima beans
			Mung beans
			Navy beans
			Peas
			Pigeon beans
			Pinto beans
			Refried beans (low-fat)
			Romano beans
			Soybeans
			Split peas

	🔴 RED LIGHT	🟡 YELLOW LIGHT	🟢 GREEN LIGHT
beverages	Alcoholic drinks (in general)	Beer**	Bottled water
	Coconut milk	Coconut milk	Club soda
	Coffee (regular)	Coffee (with skim milk, no sugar)	Decaffeinated coffee (with skim milk, no sugar)
	Fruit drinks (all)		
	Milk (whole or 2%)	Diet soft drinks (caffeinated)	Diet soft drinks (no caffeine)
	Regular soft drinks	Milk (1%)	Herbal teas
		Most fruit juices (unsweetened)	Light instant hot chocolate
	Rice milk	Red wine (one glass, preferably with dinner)**	Milk (skim)
	Sweetened juices, including naturally sweetened (all)		Soy milk (plain, low-fat)
		Vegetable juices	Tea (with skim milk, no sugar)
breads	Bagels and rolls	Crispbreads (with fiber; e.g., Ryvita High Fiber)	Crispbreads (with high fiber; e.g., Wasa Fiber)*
	Baguettes and other crusty white breads	Pita (whole wheat)	Homemade Apple Bran Muffins (see page 86)
	Biscuits	Sourdough bread	
	Cake/cookies		
	Corn bread	Tortillas (whole wheat)	Whole-grain, high-fiber bread (at least 3g fiber per slice)*
	Croissants and pastries	Whole-grain breads (less than 3g fiber/slice)	
	Croutons		
	Doughnuts		
	English muffins		
	Hamburger/ hot dog buns		
	Kaiser rolls		
	Melba toast		

*Limit serving size (see page 25).
**In Phase II, a glass of wine or an occasional beer may be included.

	● RED LIGHT	○ YELLOW LIGHT	● GREEN LIGHT
breads (continued)	Muffins (commercial) Pancakes/waffles Pizza Stuffing Tortillas (regular) White bread and other non-whole-grain sandwich bread		
cereal grains	Almond flour Amaranth Couscous Millet Polenta Rice (short-grain, white, instant) Rice cakes Rice noodles White flour	Corn Cornstarch Couscous (whole wheat) Spelt	Arrowroot flour Barley Bran (oat, wheat) Buckwheat Bulgur Gram flour Kamut (not puffed) Quinoa Rice (basmati, brown, long-grain, wild)* Wheat berries Wheat germ Whole wheat flour
cereals	All cold cereals except those listed as yellow- or green-light Cereal bars Cream of Wheat Granola	Post Shredded Wheat'N Bran	Cold cereals with at least 10g fiber or protein per serving (e.g., All-Bran, Bran Buds, Fiber One, Kashi GoLean, Kashi GoLean Crunch!)*

*Limit serving size (see page 25).

	RED LIGHT	YELLOW LIGHT	GREEN LIGHT
cereals (continued)	Granola bars (commercial) Grits Instant/quick-cook oatmeal Muesli (commercial)		Homemade Granola Bars (see page 87) Homemade Muesli (see page 64)* Kasha* Kashi GoLean hot cereal* Large-flake, rolled, or steel-cut oats (e.g., Old-Fashioned Quaker Oats)* Oat bran*
condiments/ seasonings	Barbecue sauce Croutons Honey mustard Ketchup Mayonnaise (regular) Relish Steak sauce Tartar sauce	Mayonnaise (light)	Capers Chili powder Extracts (vanilla, etc.) Garlic Gravy mix (maximum 20 calories per ¼ cup serving) Herbs/spices Horseradish Hummus Mayonnaise (fat-free) Mustard Salsa (no added sugar) Sauerkraut Soy sauce (low sodium)

*Limit serving size (see page 25).

	RED LIGHT	YELLOW LIGHT	GREEN LIGHT
condiments/ seasonings (continued)			Teriyaki sauce Vinegar (all types) Worcestershire sauce
dairy	Almond milk Cheese (regular) Chocolate milk Coconut milk Cottage cheese (whole or 2%) Cream Cream cheese (regular) Evaporated milk Goat's milk Ice cream (regular) Milk (whole or 2%) Rice milk Sour cream (regular) Yogurt (whole or 2%)	Cheese (low-fat) Cream cheese (light) Ice cream (low-fat) Milk (1%) Sour cream (light) Yogurt (low-fat with sugar)	Buttermilk (skim or 1%) Cheese (fat-free) Cottage cheese (1% or fat-free) Cream cheese (nonfat) Extra-low-fat cheese (e.g., Laughing Cow Light, Boursin Light) Flavored yogurt (fat-free with sweetener) Frozen yogurt (½ cup; low-fat) Ice cream (low-fat and no added sugar)* Milk (skim) Sour cream (fat-free or 1%) Soy cheese (low-fat) Soy milk (plain, low-fat) Soy/whey protein powder

*Limit serving size (see page 25).

	● RED LIGHT	● YELLOW LIGHT	● GREEN LIGHT
fats/nuts/ oils	Butter	Corn oil	Almonds*
	Coconut oil	Mayonnaise (light)	Canola oil*/seed
	Hard margarine	Natural nut butters	Cashews*
	Lard		Flaxseed
	Mayonnaise (regular)	Natural peanut butter (100% peanuts)	Hazelnuts*
	Palm oil	Nuts, except those listed as green-light	Macadamia nuts*
	Peanut butter (regular and light)	Peanut oil	Mayonnaise (fat-free)
	Salad dressings (bottled, regular)	Peanuts	Olive oil*
	Tropical oils	Pecans	Pistachios*
	Vegetable shortening	Salad dressings (bottled, light)	Salad dressings (low-fat, low sugar)
		Sesame oil	Soft margarine (nonhydroge- nated, light; e.g., Promise Light)*
		Soft margarine (nonhydroge- nated)	Vegetable oil sprays
		Soy oil	Vinaigrette
		Sunflower oil	
		Vegetable oil	
		Walnuts	
fruits (fresh/ frozen)	Cantaloupe	Apricots	Apples
	Honeydew melon	Bananas	Avocado (¼ of the fruit)
	Kumquats	Figs	Blackberries
	Melons	Kiwis	Blueberries
	Prunes	Mangoes	Cherries
	Watermelon	Papayas	Cranberries
		Persimmons	Grapefruit
		Pineapple	Grapes
		Pomegranates	Guavas

*Limit serving size (see page 25).

	● RED LIGHT	○ YELLOW LIGHT	● GREEN LIGHT
fruits (fresh/ frozen) (continued)			Lemons Oranges Peaches/ nectarines Pears Plums Raspberries Rhubarb Strawberries
fruits (bottled/ canned/ dried)	Applesauce containing sugar Canned fruits in syrup (all) Dates (dried)* Dried fruit (most)* Prunes Raisins*	Apricots (canned in juice) Apricots (dried)* Cranberries (dried)* Fruit cocktail in juice	Apples (dried) Applesauce (unsweetened) Fruit spreads (double fruit, no added sugar) Mandarin oranges Peaches/pears in juice
juices	Fruit drinks (all) Prune Sweetened juices, including naturally sweetened (all) Watermelon	Apple (unsweetened) Cranberry (unsweetened) Grapefruit (unsweetened) Orange (unsweetened) Pear (unsweetened) Pineapple (unsweetened) Vegetable	Eat the fruit rather than drink its juice

*You may use a modest amount of dried fruit for baking.

	● RED LIGHT	○ YELLOW LIGHT	● GREEN LIGHT
meat*/ poultry*/ seafood*/ eggs/ meat substitutes	Bacon (regular)	Beef (sirloin steak, sirloin tip)	Beef (lean cuts)
	Beef (brisket, short ribs)	Chicken thighs, wings, and legs (skinless)	Canadian bacon
	Bologna		Chicken breast (skinless)
	Bratwurst	Fish canned in oil	Deli meats (lean)
	Breaded fish and seafood	Flank steak	Egg Beaters
	Duck	Ground beef (lean—10–20% fat)	Egg whites
	Goose		Ground beef (extra lean—10% or less fat)
	Ground beef (regular—more than 20% fat)	Lamb (lean cuts)	Liquid eggs
	Hamburgers	Pork (lean cuts)	Moose
	Hot dogs	Tofu (firm)	Pastrami (turkey)
	Lamb (rack)	Turkey bacon	Pork tenderloin
	Organ meats	Turkey leg (skinless)	Rabbit
	Pastrami (beef)	Whole eggs (preferably omega-3)	Sashimi
	Paté		Seafood, fresh or frozen (no batter or breading), or canned (in water)
	Pork (back ribs, blade, spare ribs)		Smoked salmon
	Processed meats		Soy cheese (low-fat)
	Salami		Soy/whey protein powder
	Sausages		Tofu (soft)
	Sushi		Turkey breast (skinless)
			Turkey roll
			Veal
			Veggie burger
			Venison

*Limit serving size (see page 25).

	● RED LIGHT	○ YELLOW LIGHT	● GREEN LIGHT
pasta	All canned pastas Couscous Gnocchi Macaroni and cheese Noodles (canned or instant) Pasta filled with cheese and/or meat		Any shape (use whole wheat or protein-enriched if available), cooked al dente*
pasta sauces	Alfredo Canned/bottled sauces with added meat or cheese Canned/bottled sauces with added sugar or sucrose	Basil pesto Sun-dried tomato pesto	Canned/bottled sauces with vegetables (light, no added sugar; e.g., Colavita, Classico, and Healthy Choice) Homemade green-light sauces
snacks	Bagels Candy Cookies Crackers Doughnuts French fries Granola bars (commercial) Ice cream (regular) Jell-O Melba toast	Bananas Dark chocolate (70% cocoa)** Ice cream (low-fat) Nuts, except those listed as green-light Popcorn (microwave light)	Almonds* Applesauce (unsweetened) Canned peaches/pears in juice Cottage cheese (1% or fat-free) Extra-low-fat cheese (e.g., Laughing Cow Light, Boursin Light)

*Limit serving size (see page 25).
**For chocoholics only; high cocoa (70%) dark chocolate in small quantities. Treat as a concession and eat only occasionally.

	● RED LIGHT	● YELLOW LIGHT	● GREEN LIGHT
snacks **(continued)**	Muffins (commercial) Popcorn (microwave, pre-popped) Potato chips Pretzels Pudding Raisins** Rice cakes Sorbet Tortilla chips Trail mix White bread		Flavored yogurt (fat-free with sweetener) Fresh fruit (most; see page 143) Fresh vegetables (most; see page 148) Frozen yogurt (½ cup; low-fat) Hazelnuts* High-protein bars*** Homemade Apple Bran Muffins (see page 86) Homemade Granola Bars (see page 87) Ice cream (low-fat and no added sugar)* Macadamia nuts* Pickles Seeds (most; e.g., flax, pumpkin, sesame, sunflower) Soy nuts Sugar-free hard candies

*Limit serving size (see page 25).

**You may use a modest amount of dried fruit for baking.

***12 to 15 grams protein per 50- to 60-gram bar, e.g., Balance; ½ bar per serving.

	RED LIGHT	YELLOW LIGHT	GREEN LIGHT
soups	All cream-based soups Canned black bean Canned green/split pea Canned puréed vegetable	Canned chicken noodle Canned lentil Canned tomato	Canned chunky bean and vegetable (e.g., Campbell's Healthy Request) Homemade soups with green-light ingredients Miso
sugar and sweeteners	Agave nectar Corn syrup Glucose Honey Molasses Splenda Brown Sugar Blend Sugar (all types)	Fructose Sugar alcohols (e.g., maltitol, xylitol)	Equal Splenda Stevia Sugar Twin Sugar Twin Granulated Brown Sweet'N Low
vegetables (fresh/frozen)	Coleslaw (commercial) Fava beans French fries Hash browns Home fries Parsnips Potatoes (instant, mashed, or baked) Rutabagas Turnips	Artichokes Beets Corn Potatoes (boiled) Pumpkin Squash Sweet potatoes Yams	Alfalfa sprouts Asparagus Avocado (¼ of the fruit) Beans (green/wax) Bell peppers Bok choy Broccoli Broccoli rabe Brussels sprouts Cabbage (all varieties) Carrots Cauliflower

	RED LIGHT	YELLOW LIGHT	GREEN LIGHT
vegetables (fresh/ frozen) (continued)			Celery
			Collard greens
			Cucumbers
			Eggplant
			Fennel
			Garlic
			Hearts of palm
			Kale
			Kohlrabi
			Leeks
			Lettuce (all varieties)
			Mushrooms
			Mustard greens
			Okra
			Olives*
			Onions
			Peas
			Peppers (hot)
			Pickles
			Potatoes (boiled small, preferably new)*
			Radicchio
			Radishes
			Rapini
			Salad greens (all varieties)
			Snow peas
			Spinach
			Swiss chard
			Tomatoes
			Zucchini

*Limit serving size (see page 25).

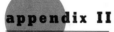

G.I. Diet Shopping List

PANTRY

baking/cooking

- [ ] Baking powder/ soda
- [ ] Cocoa (70%)*
- [ ] Dried apricots*
- [ ] Sliced almonds
- [ ] Wheat/oat bran
- [ ] Whole wheat flour

beans (canned)

- [ ] Baked beans (low-fat)
- [ ] Mixed salad beans
- [ ] Most varieties
- [ ] Vegetarian chili

bread

- [ ] Whole-grain, high-fiber (3g fiber per slice)

cereals

- [ ] All-Bran

*Use sparingly during Phase I.

- [ ] Bran Buds
- [ ] Fiber One
- [ ] Kashi GoLean
- [ ] Oatmeal (large-flake, rolled, or steel-cut)
- [ ] Soy protein powder

drinks

- [ ] Bottled water
- [ ] Club soda
- [ ] Decaffeinated coffee/tea
- [ ] Diet decaffeinated soft drinks

fats/oils

- [ ] Canola oil
- [ ] Mayonnaise (fat-free)
- [ ] Olive oil
- [ ] Salad dressings (low-fat, low sugar)
- [ ] Soft margarine (nonhydrogenated, light)
- [ ] Vegetable oil spray

fruit (canned/bottled)

- [ ] Applesauce (unsweetened)
- [ ] Mandarin oranges
- [ ] Peaches in juice
- [ ] Pears in juice

pasta (whole wheat or protein-enriched)

- [ ] Capellini
- [ ] Fettuccine
- [ ] Macaroni
- [ ] Penne
- [ ] Spaghetti
- [ ] Vermicelli

pasta sauces (vegetable-based only, light)

- [ ] Classico
- [ ] Colavita
- [ ] Healthy Choice

rice

- ☐ Basmati
- ☐ Brown
- ☐ Long-grain
- ☐ Wild

seasonings

- ☐ Flavored vinegars/sauces

- _____
- _____
- _____
- _____

- ☐ Spices/herbs

- _____
- _____
- _____
- _____

snacks

- ☐ High-protein bars (e.g., Balance)

soups

- ☐ Healthy Request

sweeteners

- ☐ Splenda, Stevia, Sugar Twin, Sweet'N Low (and other nonsugar sweeteners)

FRIDGE/ FREEZER

dairy

- ☐ Buttermilk
- ☐ Cottage cheese (1% or fat-free)
- ☐ Flavored yogurt (fat-free with sweetener)
- ☐ Frozen yogurt (nonfat)
- ☐ Ice cream (low-fat and no added sugar)
- ☐ Milk (skim)
- ☐ Sour cream (1% or fat-free)

fruit (fresh/frozen)

- ☐ Apples
- ☐ Blackberries
- ☐ Blueberries
- ☐ Cherries
- ☐ Grapefruit
- ☐ Grapes
- ☐ Lemons
- ☐ Limes
- ☐ Oranges
- ☐ Peaches
- ☐ Pears
- ☐ Plums
- ☐ Raspberries
- ☐ Strawberries

meat/poultry/ seafood/eggs

- ☐ Chicken breast (skinless)
- ☐ Egg Beaters
- ☐ Egg whites
- ☐ Ground beef (extra lean)
- ☐ Ham/turkey/chicken (lean deli)
- ☐ Liquid eggs
- ☐ Seafood, fresh or frozen (no batter or breading), or canned (in water)
- ☐ Turkey breast (skinless)
- ☐ Veal

vegetables

- ☐ Asparagus
- ☐ Beans (green/wax)
- ☐ Bell and hot peppers
- ☐ Broccoli
- ☐ Cabbage
- ☐ Carrots
- ☐ Cauliflower
- ☐ Celery
- ☐ Cucumber
- ☐ Eggplant
- ☐ Leeks
- ☐ Lettuce
- ☐ Mushrooms
- ☐ Olives
- ☐ Onions
- ☐ Pickles
- ☐ Potatoes (small, preferably new)
- ☐ Snow peas
- ☐ Spinach
- ☐ Tomatoes
- ☐ Zucchini

Dining Out and Travel Tips

	RED LIGHT	GREEN LIGHT
breakfast	Bacon/sausage Bagels Eggs Most cold cereals Muffins Pancakes/waffles	All-Bran Egg whites/Egg Beaters—omelet (no cheese, please) Egg whites/Egg Beaters—scrambled Fruit Oatmeal (not instant) Yogurt (fat-free with sweetener)
lunch	Bakery products Butter/mayonnaise Cheese Fast food Pasta-based meals Pizza/bagels Potatoes (replace with double vegetables) White bread	Lean deli meats Pasta—$\frac{1}{4}$ plate maximum Salads—low-fat (dressing on the side) Sandwiches—open-faced; whole-grain, high-fiber bread Soups—chunky vegetable and bean Vegetables Wraps—$\frac{1}{2}$ pita or low-carb tortilla, no mayonnaise

	● RED LIGHT	● GREEN LIGHT
dinner	Beef/lamb/pork Butter/mayonnaise Caesar salad Desserts—pastries, ice cream, candy Pasta-based meals Potatoes (replace with double vegetables) Soups—cream-based White bread White rice (regular)	Chicken/turkey (skinless) Fruit Pasta—¼ plate Rice (basmati, brown, long-grain, wild)—¼ plate Salads—low-fat (dressing on the side) Seafood—not breaded or battered Soups—chunky vegetable or bean Vegetables
snacks	Candy Chips (all types) Cookies/muffins Popcorn (microwave, pre-popped) Pretzels	Fat-free cottage cheese with unsweetened fruit preserves Fresh fruit ½ High-protein bar (e.g., Balance) Nuts (preferably almonds, hazelnuts, or macadamias)—8–10 Yogurt—fat-free with sweetener

PORTIONS

Meat/Fish	Palm of hand/pack of cards
Vegetables	Minimum ½ plate
Rice/Pasta	Maximum ¼ plate
Small (preferably new) potatoes	2 to 3 in Phase I; 3 to 4 in Phase II

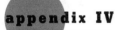

The Ten Golden G.I. Diet Rules

1. Eat three meals and three snacks every day. Don't skip meals—particularly breakfast.

2. In Phase I, stick with green-light products only.

3. When it comes to food, quantity is as important as quality. Shrink your usual portions, particularly of meat, pasta, and rice.

4. Always ensure that each meal contains a measure of carbohydrates, protein, and fat.

5. Eat at least three times more vegetables and fruit than usual.

6. Drink plenty of fluids, preferably water.

7. Stay 90 percent on the program, allowing yourself 10 percent "wiggle room." This diet is not a straitjacket.

8. Find a friend to join you for mutual support.

9. Set realistic goals. Try to lose an average of a pound a week and record your progress to reinforce your sense of achievement.

10. Don't view this as a diet. It's the basis of how you will eat for the rest of your life.

G.I. DIET WEEKLY WEIGHT/WAIST LOG

week	date	weight	waist	comments
1.				
2.				
3.				
4.				
5.				
6.				
7.				
8.				
9.				
10.				
11.				
12.				
13.				
14.				
15.				
16.				
17.				
18.				
19.				
20.				

DISHING UP DINNER

Use this diagram to compare the way we've traditionally visualized our dinner plate with the healthier G.I. Diet version.

THE TRADITIONAL
DINNER PLATE

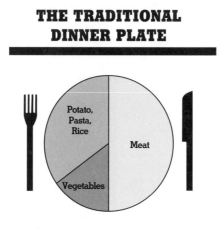

THE G.I. DIET
DINNER PLATE

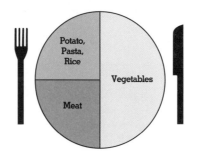

General Index

Also see the Recipe Index on pages 163–64.

To determine whether a specific food is green-light, yellow-light, or red-light, please refer to The Complete G.I. Diet on pages 138–49.

A

Abdominal fat, 19, 131, 135
Alcohol, 51, 91–92, 94, 139
  wine, 25, 51, 61, 90, 91, 93, 139
Alzheimer's disease, 4, 131, 135
Arby's, 99
Atherosclerosis, 133, 135

B

Backpack or shopping bag motivator, 53–54, 92, 121
Barbecues, 61
Baseline measurements, 54
Beans (legumes), 6, 13, 46, 52, 63, 129, 138, 150
Beef, 81, 145. *See also* Meat
  steak dinners, 82, 90
Beer, 91–92, 139
Behavior change, 107–18
  cleaning the plate and, 111–12, 115
  eating too quickly and, 110, 115
  emotional eating and, 113–15
  grazing and, 109, 115, 117
  high-sugar, high-fat treats and, 113
  not drinking enough and, 110–11
  not taking time to eat properly and, 108–9
  rewarding exercise with food and, 111
  shopping on empty stomach and, 112
  skipping breakfast and, 108
  tips for, 115–18
  unconscious eating and, 110, 116, 117

Beverages, 139, 150. *See also* Alcohol
  coffee, 32, 49–50, 89, 104, 106
  dining out and travel tips for, 104
  fruit drinks or juices, 29, 30, 50, 89, 144
  in Phase I, 48–51
  skim milk, 13, 31, 49
  tea, 32, 50
  water, 48, 49, 104, 105, 110–11, 154
Blood pressure, 96. *See also* Hypertension
Blood sugar (blood glucose), 6, 30, 51, 57, 93, 108–9, 111, 134
  Glycemic Index and, 8, 9–12
Body image, 119
Body Mass Index (BMI), 15–19, 21
Breads, 7, 25, 32, 89, 90, 150
  food charts for, 28, 34–35, 43, 139–40
  in restaurants, 105
  for sandwiches, 38, 73
Breakfast, 13
  dining out and travel tips for, 103, 152
  meal ideas for, 63–68. *See also* Recipe Index, 163
  in Phase I, 26–32, 63–68
  in Phase II, 89
  skipping, 108, 154
  taking time for, 108–9
Brown-bag lunches, 38–39
Buffets, all-you-can-eat, 100
Burger King, 98

C

Caffeine, 32, 49–50, 106
Calories, 3, 11, 20–21, 24
  food labels and, 55
  maintaining new weight and, 88–89
  in pound of body fat, 21, 125–26
Cancer, 4, 6, 19, 91, 120, 131, 132, 134–35, 136

Canola oil, 25, 62, 137
Carbohydrates, 6–8, 26, 134, 154
 in Phase I breakfast, 27–29, 34–36
 in Phase I dinner, 43–44
 in Phase I lunch, 34–36
Cereals, 8, 25, 27–28, 30–31, 89,
 140–41, 150
Cheese, 4, 31–32, 61–62
 cottage, 13, 31, 85
 yogurt, 84
Chicken, 38, 46, 97, 129, 145.
 See also Poultry
Childhood, emotional eating
 rooted in, 114–15
Children, 51–52, 102
Chinese restaurants, 24, 100
Chocolate, 25, 90–91, 113, 124
Cholesterol, 4, 91, 133
Cleaning one's plate, 111–12, 115
Clothes, as motivator, 119, 120
Coffee, 32, 49–50, 89, 104, 106
Color-coded system, 21–22,
 23–24
Comfort, eating for, 113–15, 116
Commuting, exercise and, 127
Condiments, 37, 141–42
Convenience foods, 108
Cooking techniques, 24, 60–61
Cottage cheese, 13, 31, 85
Cravings, dealing with, 123–24
Cycling, 125
 on stationary bike, 127–28

D

Dairy products, 6, 12, 13, 31–32, 63,
 129, 136, 151. *See also* Cheese;
 Milk; Yogurt
 food charts for, 27, 34, 42, 142
Dementia, 135
Desserts, 48, 93
 in restaurants, 104, 106
Diabetes, 19, 30, 113, 120, 126, 131,
 134, 135, 136
Digestive process, 3, 12, 24, 60, 63
 Glycemic Index and, 8, 9–12
Dining and driving in U.S.A., 101–5

Dinner, 13, 108–9
 dining out and travel tips for, 104,
 153
 meal ideas for, 75–84. *See also*
 Recipe Index, 163
 in Phase I, 26, 41–48, 75–84
 in Phase II, 90
Drinking enough fluids, 110–11
Drinks. *See* Beverages

E

Eating out, 96–106
 at all-you-can-eat buffets, 100
 driving in U.S.A. and, 101–5
 at ethnic restaurants, 100–101
 at family-style restaurants, 99, 102–5
 at fast-food restaurants, 96–99
 green-light options for, 99–101
 serving sizes and, 99, 102, 116
 top 10 dining tips for, 105–6
Eating slowly, 94, 105, 110
Eating too quickly, 110, 115
Eggs, 26, 27, 32, 33, 41–42, 63, 129,
 145, 151
Emotional eating, 113–15
Energy in/energy out equation, 11,
 20–21, 88–89
Energy level, 57, 119–20
 short-term fixes and, 10, 108–9
Exercise, 125–30
 health impacted by, 131, 132, 134
 losing weight and, 111, 125–26
 in Phase II, 94, 126
 rewarding with food, 111
 starting program of, 130
 strength training and, 128–29

F

Falling off wagon, 57, 93, 117, 123–24
Fast food, 96–99, 116
Fat (body), 3, 10
 abdominal, 19, 131, 135
 calories in, 21, 125–26
 estimating, 15–20
 weight loss and, 20–21
Fats, 3–5, 26, 62, 133, 134, 150, 154

Recipe Index